the
path
to your
R.E.A.L.
health

For more than 20 years I've been a client of Lunavital, Center of Integrative Medicine with services for well-being in Santiago, Dominican Republic. It's a special space that focuses on spirit, mind and body. Its eclectic and welcoming atmosphere is a reflection of Dr. Luna's passion for serving and teaching. Now you will be moved through her words and the same loving spirit that I've received at her center. Prepare your magic wand, because this book is all about you. It will guide you to take your first steps toward a renewed, healthy and invigorating life!

– JUAN PABLO CASIMIRO
Founder/CEO BIZNOVATOR

More people every day seek more than just a cure, they seek healing and that's the approach of Dr. Raquelina Luna with her R.E.A.L. therapeutic model, which shows us disease as a state of being where harmony and internal balance have been lost, and leads us to manage it on morphological, functional, psychological, energetic and spiritual planes. This book is supported by a philosophy of medicine whose aim is not to combat disease but to transmute it. It invites us to be not only healthier, but more complete.

– MARTHA BEATO
Author & Founder of Productividad y Bienestar

Each of us is responsible for our health, but this book is very helpful for finding a REAL path in the right direction, giving us a broad, clear and well-defined picture of comprehensive health. Dr. Luna is an expert guide, offering recommendations and take-home advice concerning both our lifestyle and the resources available to us through a variety of healing practices.

– MARIA CONSUELO YUNEN, MD
Founder CUTIS Clinic

Faced with the questions of those who seek healing, The Path to Your R.E.A.L. Health is an essential answer. In this work, Dr. Raquelina Luna shares her own quest and various encounters along the way. Her life becomes a reference as she accompanies any reader who chooses to embark on the journey of discovery. You can let yourself be guided through these pages with confidence in the Mysterious Force of Creation that has endowed us with the resources and capabilities to be healthy. This is a book that reminds us that we're on the path of that which is always possible and invites us to heal, love life and love each other!

– SIU LENG SANG, MD
Director, Neijing School of Chinese Medicine.

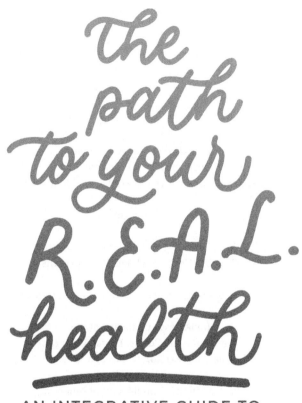

the path to your R.E.A.L. health

AN INTEGRATIVE GUIDE TO YOUR TOTAL WELL-BEING

DR. RAQUELINA LUNA

Translated & Edited by Edward Morgan

1st Edition
Published by Luna Vital Corp
Brookyn, NY

ISBN: 978-9945-8-0382-2 (Spanish edition)
ISBN: 978-0-578-78839-5 (ebook, English translation)

Library of Congress Control Number - 2020920933

Book Design: Julissa Batista
Translator and Editor: Edward Morgan
Spanish Text Editor: Roxana Amaro

Printed in the United States of America.

Published by Luna Vital Corp.
Brooklyn, NY

For more information: luna.raquelina@gmail.com

Dedicated to the REAL in you,
the love and light that you are.
Light that unites us as brothers and sisters.
To that part of us that creates a transformative field that supports,
encourages, accompanies and allows me to say:
If you heal, I heal.

TRANSLATOR'S NOTE

It's been a labor of love to translate and edit this English version of *El Camino a tu Salud R.E.A.L.* The goal was to preserve the conversational quality of the book while helping to streamline and clarify the narrative. We've made significant changes in the process and I'm indebted to Dr. Luna for her willingness, her vision and her trust.

EDWARD MORGAN
November, 2020

CONTENTS

PREFACE   *xi*

INTRODUCTION   1

PART I
REAL PREMISES

CHAPTER 1. This is about You   10

CHAPTER 2. Step from the Role of the Victim   13

CHAPTER 3. Take up your Magic Wand   16

CHAPTER 4. Seek Help   19

CHAPTER 5. An Integrative View of Health   21

CHAPTER 6. The Art of Prevention   25

CHAPTER 7. Health and Sickness   27

CHAPTER 8. The R.E.A.L. Therapeutic Model   35

PART II
REVIEW

CHAPTER 9. Review: Your History is You   44

CHAPTER 10. The Systemic Approach to Physical Health   55

CHAPTER 11. Integrating Mind, Body and Emotions   61

CHAPTER 12. Embracing your Body   72

CHAPTER 13. Correspondences in the Body   84

PART III
REMOVE

CHAPTER 14. Remove: Bet on a Detoxified Life   94
CHAPTER 15. Physical Detoxification   96
CHAPTER 16. Fasting as a Way of Purifying   103
CHAPTER 17. Toxins in your Environment   107
CHAPTER 18. The Mental and Emotional Purge   111
CHAPTER 19. The Grief in Sickness   115
CHAPTER 20. Digital Detox   118

PART IV
REPAIR

CHAPTER 21. Repair: Awaken your Gift Of Regeneration   124
CHAPTER 22. Telomeres, Live Longer and Better   130
CHAPTER 23. The Art of Eating Well   139
CHAPTER 24. Sugar!   145
CHAPTER 25. Deep Rest   151
CHAPTER 26. My Experience with Cancer   157

PART V
REVITALIZE

CHAPTER 27. Revitalize: Light up your Life   174
CHAPTER 28. You are Energy   177
CHAPTER 29. Concerning Stress   184
CHAPTER 30. More Exercise, more Health!   198
CHAPTER 31. Breathe Life   203

PART VI
RESIGNIFY

CHAPTER 32. Resignify: Discover New Colors   210

CHAPTER 33. Contemplative Tools   214

CHAPTER 34. Choose to Live in Gratitude   226

EPILOGUE   233

ACKNOWLEDGMENTS   235

APPENDIX I   237

APPENDIX II   245

NOTES   247

PREFACE

I met Raquelina several years ago when she was introduced to me at an event I was offering in Colombia. From that moment on, I knew I was facing a vanguard educator, a woman who is a leader and pioneer in health and true well-being. It was very refreshing for me to see that being a medical doctor who graduated from a traditional university, she had then gone through diverse disciplines of healing which come from different cultures populating this planet.

And I saw that she did it with an open mind and a great passion for serving and helping people, without dogmas or prejudices.

Being part of today's lifestyle, where we are bombarded all the time with much more information than we can process and living in a world full of stressful news, Dr. Raquelina Luna gave birth to this book that I view like a map.

It's a very clear guide with simple steps to learn, so that the reader, knows how to prevent and maintain his or her health or correct what's necessary to achieve the physical, mental and emotional well-being they seek and desire.

They say that when we are born, no one gives us a user manual to know how our body works or how to live our life to its fullest potential. Well, now we have it!

This book performs several very important functions. On the one hand, it gives us practical methods and elements to correct what's affecting our health, and on the other hand, it gives us that education that none of us have received in school.

How does our body work?
What do you need to perform in an excellent manner?
What's affecting my body?
What makes my body sick?
How do we make the necessary corrections?

This is what I call, "education for life!"

– LUIS DÍAZ.
Author of the best-seller: *La Memoria en las Células,
Cómo Sanar Nuestros Patrones de Conducta
(Memory in Cells, How to Heal our Behavior Patterns).*

INTRODUCTION

My name is Raquelina Luna and my life's work is to help people who want to make physical and emotional changes in order to transform what happens to them. I help lead them to change in a more conscious way. I apply my work through the body, the emotions and the mind, knowing that they're all actually one thing and that the health we desire comes when they are in balance. Over the years I've gradually changed the modality of my work. I've found a way to offer an ever more integrated approach to treatment with an expanding array of tools and a growing understanding of health. My goal is to support those who want to achieve a quality of life with a higher level of health, vitality and happiness.

This book is the culmination of my experiences. It's a compilation of many years' work and exploration through which I hope to reach a larger audience, to continue sowing seeds of consciousness in pursuit of individual well-being.

At an early age I began a personal quest that led me to an understanding of our being as spiritual and transcendent. At the same time, I pursued a formal education and graduated as a Doctor of Medicine in 1990. After graduating, I continued to research and broaden my training in a more holistic way, incorporating resources now considered as part of integrative medicine. For the last 25 years, I've been the founding director of Lunavital, an integrative health clinic in my hometown of Santiago, Dominican Republic.

From there I've traveled my country and the world, continuing my training and applying what I've learned. *The Path to Your R.E.A.L. Health* is largely a summary of all I've incorporated into my life through work on myself and through my professional practice. One way or another, like a skein of many-colored threads, the story of my career and my personal healing and transformation have been woven together. I've also gradually incorporated the psychotherapeutic tools I now apply in private consultations and with participants of workshops and conferences that I lead. So I've connected my two passions: the world of the psychological and the physical.

While studying medicine, I particularly enjoyed physiology. I was fascinated to learn about the body and its functions, the biological, chemical and electrical processes and so on. At the same time, I had a passion for human behavior, for feelings and the study of energy. I wanted to look at the body and also the intangible, which expresses itself through emotions and through something even more transcendent. Over time it grew ever clearer to me that both sides were integrated, because there is no emotion without biology and behind every particular physical imbalance is an emotional imbalance, either conscious or unconscious. I look back now and realize that my different interests opened doors for me. They led me toward an understanding that was inclusive and receptive, with space enough for polarities and space to make connections.

These days I help people to release physical or emotional pain, to embark on their journey of transformation, to reconcile and re-signify their history. I help them connect with their potential, with their own resources, empowering them to resolve what they need to resolve. Each of us holds the power of true transformation in our own hands. It's a choice we can make, a goal we can achieve, to be conscious, to set forth on a path whose destination is to be R.E.A.L. This book will help you map the route.

We live in an ideal time for a paradigm shift regarding health, a time to begin to empower ourselves, to become the drivers, to hold the reins of our own processes, our suffering, our pains, our experiences, our circumstances and our histories. Given that we live in a changing and more open world, a world of accelerated and instant communication, it's also an ideal time for us to use more tools, tools that allow us to see ourselves as complete and integral and to stop perceiving ourselves as a collection of disjointed pieces. This is the perfect moment for a shift in perception.

The big picture, the totality, means having a perspective that unifies all that happens in the body. It means connecting what happens in the organs with the processes that originate in the depths of the heart, in the mind and from the workings of the unconscious. And here's what I find synchronous and even magical. Whenever I'm able to integrate things, either by looking at myself or having the privilege of working with someone else and seeing it together, I'm amazed and awe-struck at the perfection of creation. I'm speechless in the face of what I believe to be truly providential and beyond scientific explanation.

To relieve pain, improve a condition or help stabilize an imbalance is an excellent goal. It's what anyone would want if their life was at risk or if they were simply in a state of discomfort, whether physical, mental or emotional. But to be able to go further, to see the origin, to see where a wound was conceived, from whence the unconscious program springs, to investigate other parts of our lives, to be able to regenerate in a different way; this is a leap that empowers us. It enables us to assume a more conscious lifestyle. Yes, it's truly a leap to set forth on one's own exploration, toward change, toward healing. And it's even better still when we can do preventive work. That's actually the highest goal in this vision of health.

To put it simply, the idea is to enter into a space of contact with oneself, of commitment to one's own pain and at the same time to one's own well-being. This goes far beyond merely living a "healthy" lifestyle (without appreciating it), beyond being an avid fan of fitness or eating a "lite" diet or taking up a particular spiritual practice. It requires information, so that we know ourselves better, how we function and how our parts relate. It requires us to pay attention to the body's warnings, to the language our bodies use through sensations and through physical metaphors that we can learn to interpret. It requires us to be more present with what happens here and now. It requires a change of consciousness.

In that space of consciousness everything is amplified and interconnected. We begin to understand what is happening to us and why we feel pain. Instead of an enemy that we hope to quickly escape, our pain transforms into an ally from whom we can learn another lesson and heal. Unfortunately or fortunately, many of us have to get sick, fall down, stumble, suffer or enter into conflict in order to begin to change. Or sometimes we need particular experiences to move into other levels of understanding, to transcend something and arrive where we want and need to be. This is what happened to me. When my first draft of this book was almost complete, life invited me in a forceful way to examine something further. I was diagnosed with a medullary thyroid carcinoma, a rare and typically aggressive type of cancer. My biopsy results indicated that it had begun to metastasize in my cervical ganglia.

I gave myself permission to express all the emotions that accompany a diagnosis like that. I allowed myself to experience the pain, fear, deep sadness, anger and anguish and all the feelings that rushed in on me. I didn't deny them,

I didn't try to avoid or ignore them. Instead, I let them pass through my body. I became a "body of pain" and gave myself permission to be present with all the reactions that at that moment were my teachers. This helped carry me through the arc of emotion to the other polarity where I found confidence, serenity and love.

I told myself, "Now you have the opportunity to respond to this in the same way you've taught others." I heeded the message of my biology. I transformed the disease into an experience to grow and heal parts of me that had been voiceless, parts that my body revealed to me through cancer. Trusting, I surrendered to what it was and so I was ready to take the necessary steps to come to a resolution.

I followed my own program and passed through each of the five steps I've developed and identified as **R.E.A.L.** This means I **Reviewed** my history and **Removed** toxins at every level. I "prepared the ground", giving space to my body and my emotions to begin to **Repair**. In every possible way, I **Revitalized**. And I did all this within the framework of changing my point of view to **Resignify,** to find the clues that would show me the way back to my essential being. Fortunately, in that transition to healing, I felt strengthened and more vital. I felt a deeper authenticity and more motivation than ever to share my work.

This is the method I'll share with you throughout this book. The R.E.A.L. system offers **R**esources that **E**mpower you for **A**uthenticity and self-**L**oyalty. It's about helping you create the life you deserve. It's designed so you can understand and follow the process of achieving optimal health, step by step, chapter by chapter, with the book as a guide.

The process can be very profound, depending on your ability to see or interconnect. The body can become a metaphor, a guide or a map. You always have the opportunity to examine and to interpret yourself, to do your own investigation and exploration, using the research of experts as a reference, but at the same time discovering your own resonances. And if what I've written here leaves you curious enough to start your own exploration and, at the very least, you begin to ask these kinds of questions, then I'm satisfied. The most important thing for me now is to be able to transmit all that's been fundamental in my self-healing and professional development. I want to share these experiences with those who may think that change is impossible or those who've searched but haven't been able to resolve what's happened to them. I want to share with those who identify with this kind of thinking, who might find confirmation of their knowledge and perhaps encounter something more. And I want to address those waiting for a miracle to happen from the outside or waiting for others to "heal them" without realizing that the possibility is in their own hands. I intend to link all of the levels of being and how they interconnect between the body, emotions, the energy and the mind, starting from the origin, the family, heredity and early experiences. I hope you choose to heal, which is your birthright. I hope you take the path to your true self.

Throughout the book, in addition to developing a simple theory and sharing some of my experiences, I also include a series of suggestions at the end of each chapter so that through related exercises you can internalize what you've learned and put it immediately into practice. This way you can be consistent, because healing is action.

I can assure you that change is possible. I have experienced it in myself and in many with whom I've worked. I assure you, you can connect with the committed, sane adult, the source of wisdom inside you, with your R.E.A.L. center where love resides and where you are perfect just as you are. And from there you can give yourself permission to change. I don't say this with the arrogance of one who believes anything is possible, but from the conviction that we've been endowed with the possibility of being creative with love by that Immeasurable Force that brought us together on this planet at this moment of existence, to share. The love that creates us is the same love that heals us.

I hope that you feel accompanied on this journey and that you can discover within you the power you have to love yourself, to be authentic, to be self-loyal, and to live with the consistency of putting into practice all that you learn and all that resonates in you.

Jaquelina Luna

JANUARY. 2019

I've walked a lot to learn what I know. I've traveled a lot, teaching and sharing what I know. I've taken many routes and I've also gone astray. I've lost my way and I've found it again. The most important journey has been to connect with my R.E.A.L. being where love resides and where everything becomes possible.

RAQUELINA LUNA

PART I

REAL PREMISES

**AUTHENTIC WISDOM
ALWAYS INCLUDES
SOME PREMISE OF UTILITY.**

JOSÉ LUIS RODRÍGUEZ JIMÉNEZ

CHAPTER 1

THIS IS ABOUT YOU

"The patient is his own best doctor and the doctor,
his companion."

— PARACELSUS

What I'm proposing here is the renewal of an old approach to health in which you become the prime mover. You lead your own process. Take charge as an adult, responsible for your own well-being. And when you need help, you seek it out. Because you know what? This is about you and your health. I believe in the power of personal responsibility, of choosing to make things happen.

From the earliest days of my spiritual search I learned that I was responsible for myself and that no one else could accomplish anything for me. Just as no one can eat for me, no one can make the changes I need to make. No one can think or feel for me. No one can forgive for me or give me peace of mind. I learned that, like everyone else, I own my own process.

This is also true about health. Every adult human being is responsible for their own health, their well-being, their own care. Therapists, doctors and healers of all kinds intervene simply as companions. We support to the extent that another person can. We suggest, educate and guide. But it's the patient's job to do the real work. Obviously, we prepare, we bring our knowledge and put it at the service of the patient. But there's no way a doctor can do the work for anyone else: the transformative power is within you. You are responsible for making your own life changes and movements, from your consciousness, at whatever level you are now. I think understanding this is critical before we delve into more specific topics.

It's extremely valuable to surrender to a therapeutic process, but right now I'm sharing the other side of that coin. In my experience, it's often the case that a patient consulting with a professional just wants to put the process into that person's hands. Take care of me! Take this away from me, just do whatever! The patient doesn't ask, doesn't question and doesn't look deeper. They don't think of the process as belonging to them or that most of the healing is up to them. Trust is fine, but when you leave everything in someone else's hands, it's as if whatever follows is alien to you and belongs to the doctor, psychologist or therapist. Until you apply yourself, nothing much can happen; real change isn't possible because it depends on someone else. The *magic* happens when you take over and begin to apply yourself from wherever you are, from whatever options exist for you (e.g. by quitting a habit, changing your diet, getting up early to exercise). Then your energy shifts. As you incorporate that change into your life, you become more receptive to a healing process.

There are also those who seek quick, miraculous solutions and who react to the measures proposed by a professional as if they were punishment, sacrifice or simply impossible.

Then there are others who know it all. They've researched everything, they know all the theories and dispute absolutely everything that's proposed to them. Moreover, they demand guarantees. The extremes in these cases are a hindrance to balanced support.

I'm asking something here that might shock you. Do you really want to heal? Is your energy available and committed to your healing? Because deep down, though it may seem incredible, despite expressing a strong desire to heal and showing up for every appointment, many people don't make a real commitment or show a true willingness to get better. You may understand this more fully when we tackle the concept of the unconscious, where we store many of our *whys*.

Many people seeking help just want to be told what to do. They need to be given all the energy. They need a miracle that comes from outside, so throughout the process their own energy remains passive. This is what prevails in our current health culture.

It's also true that those of us who work as healers need to have our lives in order. We also need help, we need to work on ourselves and understand our own situation in order to be of service to others. I had to learn to help myself and heal my own story first, so I could work with my patients and their stories from a better place, respecting their processes but also setting healthier and more balanced boundaries.

The job of a professional is to actively listen and direct questions, to suggest, to accompany your journey of discovery, to help guide you toward well-being through increasingly better health as far as you can go. But it depends on you accessing your own power. The therapist is responsible for a minimal part of the success of any therapy. Swallowing a pill, using a medicinal plant, having acupuncture sessions or any other treatment is not enough, in my opinion. You have to get involved, integrate and take charge of your process in pursuit of your well-being.

Open your mind to the possibilities. Healing requires a commitment to yourself and to change. Many people have done it. To achieve different results, you need to behave differently. It all begins by thinking differently.

CHAPTER 2

STEP FROM THE ROLE OF THE VICTIM

"When you stop playing the victim and start being a learner your life starts to change for the better."

— ENRIC CORBERA

Behind that first untaken step toward healing often lies an excuse masquerading as a victim. You can be a victim in many ways: the victim of a disease, the victim of a relationship, the victim of a work situation, an economic crisis and on and on. When you enter into victimhood you go round and round without going anywhere.

We are not victims of life, of sickness, of other people or of the past. Whether it's conscious or unconscious, there's always a degree of responsibility that's ours and, as we begin the journey of healing, this is what we have to face. It doesn't matter where you start, there's always something you can do. And once you do it you've taken the first step.

Likewise, when we have conflict in our interpersonal relationships, we tend to place responsibility outside of ourselves by blaming the other person. Yet in every situation, whether you realize it or not, there's a shared responsibility. The movement begins when you can look at yourself and take care of the percentage of things that belong to you, taking responsibility without guilt. That's working from the inner adult.

Lodged in the inner child of many adults is a sense of blame or personal guilt that holds us back from the possibility of greater health. This blaming of self or others is deeply related to the conscious or unconscious blaming of those who gave us our lives: our parents. And, depending on the context, we extend this feeling outward to our partner, our children, our friends and our community. When we mature and become adults beyond mere chronology, we leave behind our childhood grievances and move on. This means we're able to say to ourselves, "Whatever others don't give me, I can give myself."

When you realize something and then integrate it with love, you can heal. New and important realizations become possible when your heart opens. You see connections and many of your conditions begin to make sense at the physical, mental or emotional level. This opening takes you out of playing the victim and being lazy. It connects you to an understanding of the process, of what you can do for yourself. This recognition brings you closer to self-responsibility and to compassion.

When we get new information or tap into something true or suddenly a lightbulb goes on, the thing to do is respond. Do something concrete and act in coherence with your new perspective. Otherwise, the process remains an unproductive theory. It becomes sterile. Remember that healing comes with action. So take the first step on this R.E.A.L. path!

ACTIONS FOR A R.E.A.L. LIFE

Think of a difficult situation in your life regarding a relationship with someone else. Think of something you see as accidental or impossible to change because it's caused by the other person or circumstances outside your control.

Ask yourself:

In what way have I contributed for this to happen?

What part of me needs this lesson and attracts it?

What does this symptom or disease reveal to me?

What is my need for this person to show me this? (For example: to hurt me, take me for granted, lie to me, ignore me, deceive me, betray me, etc.)

When did this happen to me before?

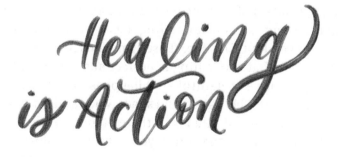

CHAPTER 3

TAKE UP YOUR MAGIC WAND

*"Magic is a bridge that allows you to go from the visible world
to the invisible. And learn the lessons of both worlds."*
— PAULO COELHO

In the early years of my search, I learned that we all have
an inner magician and we all have the power to transform,
to continually realign ourselves and move toward a better
life.

When I say "magic wand," I'm referring of course to the
storied wands of wizards. I'm not referring to the *fantasy
magic* promises of instant results that abound in the current health market. I'm not selling the idea of instant transformation or anything like, "Lose 10 pounds in seven days!"
nor the idea that everything is perfect and wonderful and
nothing negative or painful ever happens. In this world of
polarities there's both light and shadow, joy and sorrow.

The magic wand alludes to the metaphor of the magician within you and the ability you have to transform pain
and shadows to produce change, as opposed to giving your
power away. And it's not a matter of time. The point is to go
through the process while simultaneously, magically opening ourselves. A magician is in touch with his or her inner
strength and yet also knows how to actively wait for the

process to unfold. A magician waits with a certainty that they can achieve a genuine purpose when they act with the humility of knowing they're part of a higher order that sustains them.

Magic happens when you choose to interact with the universe around you and use your power in a transcendent way. It's given when you're in touch with your gifts and resources and confident in your worth, while also trusting and yielding to that Higher Order we call God, Creator or Great Spirit.

Connecting with this inner magician means remembering and recognizing who you are. It means connecting with the truth, love and the simplicity of that which is essential. To the extent that we forget who we are and move away from authenticity, we lose our creative power, our vision and our sense of worth. Then we begin to betray our own destiny. Our magic is lost in fear like a forgotten toy in a deep, dark trunk that's filled with anxiety.

Magic is inherent in our nature, in our essential humanity. The primary way to access it is by recovering the innocence of our inner children, entering that authentic, original part of us which is still intact, no matter all the conditioning or years that have passed in a kind of exile. That part of us has no self-doubt and still has dreams and visions. For that inner child anything is possible: to live in dreams, in surprise, in the magical moment. This is the part of us that relishes the present, right now, because there's nothing else.

You may feel something's missing in your life. Or a sense of failure. Maybe you feel incomplete. You're not truly happy but you settle for a status quo you don't really want and doesn't fulfill you. You're living a life that doesn't excite you, where you just go through the motions. This is living in fear, the opposite of living in magic. But knowing that nothing is wasted or lost in the universe, your magical soul is quite capable of transforming fear into love. You can become a great recycler.

The more coherent you are, the more aligned and centered, the more you remember who you truly are and reconcile with that reality, the more you'll be alert to the signs and clearly see the path. Like the Magi – the Three Wise Men – you'll be guided by the perfect star and travel unerringly to the birthplace of love. And there, you'll give yourself the gifts of incense, gold and myrrh.

Capitalize on life with joy, intelligence and love and travel your own unique road of learning. I acknowledge your power. I give you back your magic wand.

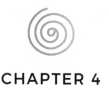

CHAPTER 4

SƐƐK HƐLP

"Helping others is an art. Like all art, it requires a skill that one can learn and exercise. It also requires empathy with the person who comes in search of help. That is to say, it requires an understanding of what is right for that person and at the same time transcends and orients them toward a more global context."

— BERT HELLINGER

The title of this chapter might seem to contradict the previous chapters, but to seek help while recognizing one's own responsibility is quite healthy. It's actually a sign of strength to acknowledge the need for help. It shows determination and a desire for change.

In the medical world, the need to ask for help is more understood and more of a given. In a physical crisis we know that we need help, so we seek out an expert.

Of course, all of us go through pain and suffering and sometimes these are overwhelming. Other times they're intense, long-lasting experiences which cause us to lose focus, perspective and even hope. But there are also other, not quite desperate moments when we lose our perspective and we're confused. We realize that we're repeating patterns or situations and we need to re-direct our lives. And though many times it's thanks to a crisis that we move forward (because the signs become impossible to ignore), we don't need to have symptoms to seek help. We don't need to be sick, in conflict or in the midst of profound suffering. It's enough to feel the need for change, to want to prevent illness on a deeper level or to simply want to live on a different level of consciousness. In all of these situations, it's valid to seek whatever professional help you need, to look for someone who can lend you some aid and help you find the right tools, skills and resources that you have within you.

Naturally, I'm assuming that the person seeking help is an adult, an equal consulting another equal. And I'm assuming the professional doesn't treat that person like a child, assuming responsibilities for them that they should take on for themselves. This also implies that the patient doesn't settle for childish solutions. If these premises are clear to both parties, help can flow between them in a balanced way.

Ask and you shall be given. When we're ready, the teacher appears in a timely manner.

CHAPTER 5

AN INTEGRATIVE VIEW OF HEALTH

*"The true journey of discovery is not about taking new paths,
but about having new eyes."*

– MARCEL PROUST

Integrative medicine or integrative health springs from the concept that the human being is composed of a physical body, an emotional body, a mental body, an energetic or vital body and a spiritual body. All of these are interconnected and interdependent. So although to study and understand them we look at them separately, it's impossible to separate them. This approach is multidimensional and this is how I've worked for 26 years.

The holistic approach goes beyond being either unconventional or conventional because it's more than just a particular technique or therapy. When we talk about integrative medicine or health we are generally referring to the fusion of conventional, mainstream or official medicine (also called allopathic) with more natural, energetic and less invasive resources, albeit with well-established, safe criteria. These resources are also called complementary or sometimes "alternative" medicine, though this last term is used to refer to all sorts of things.

Integrative medicine is practiced by doctors who embrace both perspectives and take the best of each.

On one hand we can view integration as the inclusion of both modalities. On the other, we can view it as the choice to perceive and work with each being as a whole, a perfect coordination of energy, body, mind, emotions and spirit. A unique entity, with a unique history, unrepeatable and complete.

For me, the great contributions of mainstream medicine are indisputable, particularly regarding the invaluable role it plays in medical intervention. I applaud and admire all that's been accomplished through medical advances and the use of technologies that add to the promise of a longer life with greater possibilities.

When it comes to the body's own resources, however, and stimulating its capacity to reconnect and balance – especially with chronic diseases – I prefer an integrative approach. This includes tools such as nutrition, phytotherapy, acupuncture, chelation, various serum therapies, body therapies, homeopathy, osteopathy, ozone therapy and energy therapies, to name a few. The goal of each of these is the recovery of our natural biological conditions. Their purpose is further aimed at recovering and maintaining health by fortifying the body and restoring its capacity for self-regulation according to its physiological design.

The same goes for psychology. I have great respect for official clinical intervention. But my inclusive nature has led me to explore and utilize other tools less recognized by the academy but which nevertheless have been validated by results. And I say this not only from knowing them as a therapist, but also though having experienced them as a patient and having achieved results in exponential leaps.

These are the psychological resources with which I'm most familiar: bioenergy, transactional analysis, clinical psychosomatics, bioneuroemotion, neurolinguistic programming, regenerative hypnotic techniques, family systemic or constellation therapy, gestalt, emotional release techniques and transgenerational approaches. All of these resources direct us back to the core, to events recorded deep in the unconscious and beyond the "obvious" facts. Naturally, they're all different models and some fit a given individual better than others. Likewise, some fit better at different stages of life experience.

These new models don't oppose conventional psychology. On the contrary, both can enrich each other and open up a world of possibilities. And again, this applies not only to a person in crisis or in need of help because of their symptoms. It also applies to those who want to prevent future crises. It applies to those who want to deepen themselves, to get to know others better or strengthen their relationships. It applies to those who want a more open perspective or simply to manage their everyday lives with more resources for empowerment.

As for conventional medicine, with a few exceptions, the prevailing hospital medical system treats each part of the body in isolation or as fragmented. It looks at correlations mostly from a biological point of view. It will take a lot of education and a huge effort to align official medical practice with integrative humanism and steer the course of health toward that new paradigm. But eventually, hopefully, we'll have a systemic change in therapeutic approaches, especially concerning prevention.

An integrated vision of health leads to a change in the definition of what it means to be healthy, well beyond the mere absence of symptoms.

None of this is new. In centuries past, many ancestral cultures developed a complementary definition of health. These are old concepts readapted to our era, enriched by research and new tools that have emerged in response to better communication and the urgent needs of the present for a change of consciousness.

In a world educated in orthodoxy, I'm advocating something that clearly represents a substantial change in how we envision the human being and how we envision therapy.

CHAPTER 6

THE ART OF PREVENTION

"Before the omen appears, it is easy to take preventive measures. What is still soft melts easily. What is still small is easily dispersed. Take care of things when they are still forming, put things in order before confusion recommences."

— TAO TE CHING

When I started studying traditional Chinese medicine (TCM), I loved hearing the story of how, until the 20th century, a Chinese village doctor was paid to keep people healthy. The doctor would visit their homes, check on their health, give prescriptions and preventive advice, monitor their diet and other habits and keep an eye on the circumstances of each family member. This doctor/counselor/therapist also knew the family's history and its tendencies and so could be very thorough concerning prevention. But when anyone got sick, the doctor's fees were withdrawn until they were well again. Clearly, the primary focus was prevention.

In this era, we're a long way from real preventive health and our basic measures of primary care have nothing to do with this ancient concept. Certainly, our general living conditions, hygiene and environmental safety have changed and largely improved. To a significant degree, they help control infections and the great historical epidemics. But in other respects, things are worse. We've polluted our environment and much of what we consume as food. We've lost the coherence of living in harmony with nature and our prevailing daily lifestyle is fundamentally unhealthy. Little by little, our consciousness is expanding, yet most people still don't really value their health until they've either lost it completely or it's too debilitated to recover. This is evident in the high and rising morbidity rates of catastrophic, degenerative diseases. And those diseases, which aren't caused by external factors, are largely preventable. Or at least they can be minimized.

Throughout this book, much of what I'm sharing is valid as prevention, especially when the changes we make to restore our health become everyday habits. It's an open invitation to you to see what you can incorporate into your lifestyle to support a healthier, fuller and happier life.

Essentially, the art of prevention is simply the art of living. It's the dynamic, ongoing recognition and expression of yourself as a multi-dimensional being in intimate communion with nature. It translates into everyday actions that nourish all that you are with what's best for you.

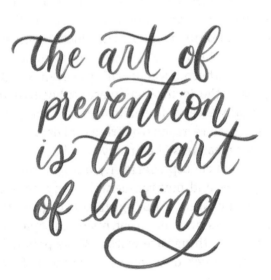

CHAPTER 7

HEALTH AND SICKNESS

*"Illness is a nuisance, and at the same time a door
that your unconscious opens for you to a happier life."*

– ADOLFO DÍAZ

Given the fascinating assembly of gears that is the human being, it follows that the situations that arise in the realm of health are likewise enriched and supplemented when addressed in a multi-dimensional way. The fact is, our body functions as a whole, interconnected within itself and with the surrounding environment. So when there's a diseased part of the body, it's not just that one part that's sick. It's the declaration of an imbalance in the whole physical system that's revealed in a particular symptom or illness.

This concept first resonated with me at age 17, when I began to delve into the philosophical aspects of my personal search. It inspired me further when I started medical school and read Hippocrates, the father of medicine. He clearly saw the interactions of body, mind and emotions as interdependent variables.

In the view of energy medicine, unbalanced emotions alter the natural flow of *qi (chi)* or vital energy and upset the balance of the internal organs, causing disease on the physical level. This can also happen in reverse. In TCM medicine the emotions, internal organs and mind-body unity all interact with each other. These are ancient concepts, written in texts such as the *Nei Jing-Sowen (The Yellow Emperor's Book of Internal Medicine)*, which dates from 1400 BC. I'm respectful of all that's been developed in the evolution of medicine and its more organicist approach (i.e. focusing on the internal organs). I appreciate that specialties exist and fulfill their function. Every day we need better-prepared doctors in many areas with sound academic preparation. However, if the doctors in any one specialty were to look beyond what specifically concerns them to see the whole, to see what might be happening elsewhere or what's behind the immediate issue, it would revolutionize the field of medicine.

The same could be said about psychologists, counselors, psychotherapists, dentists; in short, all of the specialized areas for treating the human being. It's a matter of taking into consideration the internal relationships and each part's connection to the whole. It means seeing the body itself as a system and at the same time seeing its connection with the emotions, the mind and the family.

For example, if you work on a person's teeth (or kidney or whatever), you're not simply working on that single piece of the body. You're touching deep sensitivities because the connections are complex. Likewise, if I work with a family member, I'm working on the entire family. It means moving beyond a reductive examination of only one small section and seeing the larger context.

In order to understand and further our collective process of transformation, we need to apply this vision of interconnectedness to more global, planetary and social concerns. The garbage I throw out and the water I waste or contaminate affects me and everyone else. Nothing is completely separate from me, so healing also means caring for my environment.

Returning to the body, Dr. Deepak Chopra, in his book, *The Perfect Health*, says that medicine will take a quantum leap when it contemplates the body like a river in a state perpetual change instead of like a frozen sculpture. He also points out that health is the natural state of the human being and that, along with the physical, we should include spiritual well-being in our definition. "Health is a state in which the person feels the joy and enthusiasm of living every moment, a sense of fulfillment and an awareness of harmony with the universe around it."[1]

According to the World Health Organization (WHO), health is not simply the absence of disease but a much broader totality. Since 1948, the WHO has defined health as, "a state of complete physical, mental and social well-being and not only the absence of disease or infirmities."[2]

When we look at a person and evaluate their health, we look at their relationship with themselves, their environment, their obstacles and how they react to and overcome those obstacles. In other words, we look at how they're advancing in life, how they love themselves and how they extend their love beyond themselves.

To be healthy requires that we review repetitive, unbalanced or limiting thoughts and stagnant, unexpressed or unrecognized emotions. It requires that we review the way we live, work and balance our work and rest, as well as how we manage relationships, commitments and priorities. It requires that we review the consistency between what we think, feel and do and that we are aligned with our purpose and our passions, as well as our sense of living in joy and fullness in the present.

"The state of health cannot be fully achieved," say Rüediger Dahlke and Thorwald Dethlefsen in *Illness as a Path*, "because it is not an immovable goal, just as nothing that is authentic remains still, everything flows. However, every flow contains a rhythm and the important thing is that everyone finds their own. Everyone is different, so there are no general rules for everyone. It's important to listen to oneself and there you will find the laws of life and health."[3]

Given this perspective, there's no way for anyone else to provide us with health because it involves much more than just symptoms. In any case, a doctor can provide a cure and yet not heal.

I remember when I first encountered this distinction. In 1991, I was a student in a seminar taught by Dr. José Luis Padilla, founding teacher of the Neijing School, which is dedicated to the international teaching of TCM. Dr. Padilla first explained the Chinese ideogram of healing (an ideogram is a pictographic symbol). Explaining each of the symbol's lines in turn, he showed us the difference between healing and curing. I was shocked when he said a person could die healthy. The purpose of healing, he told us, is not to keep people from dying, it is to help them enter into a consciousness of true health. I understood this intellectually, but it took a while to truly digest what he meant.

Dr. Padilla then showed us the curing ideogram and explained how a being that has entered a path of awakening can stop with the mere disappearance of symptoms or the manifested physical illness. They're cured.

Or, depending on their internal process, their cure could be just a first step on a path that might take them much further, to a state of healing.

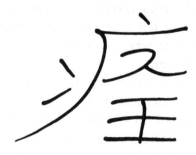

THE CURING IDEOGRAM

The healing ideogram starts with a "vertical man," which alludes to our celestial or divine origin. The man enters the circular motion of life and awakens to a consciousness of his smallness. From that place of humility and even vulnerability, he can recover coherence. Hence knowing himself as human, the man enters into his heritage as a universal being and a testimony of the celestial.

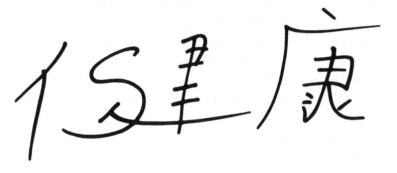

THE HEALING IDEOGRAM

To heal, then, is to reconcile life itself in your being, to live in coherence with who you are in all the areas of your life, reconciled with your lights and your shadows. To heal is to flow in connection with a greater force, following a life-purpose and a mission that's aligned with one's essence. And to get there, people often need to get sick. Sickness is actually a great opportunity!

This reinforces the aforementioned concept that the doctor or therapist is just a companion for part of the process, because the whole process depends on the individual in the intimacy of solitude.

Knowing this, the next time you receive a therapy (any therapy, whether natural or not), I encourage you to give yourself permission to be actively involved. This is what makes the difference. As I've said, it's about you. Your life changes when you change.

In that same vein, when a disease appears, it comes to show us the way. It appears as a messenger who brings us information about what we're not seeing. It speaks in metaphorical language to point out the rut we're in.

Sickness is our teacher and if we can appreciate it as such it opens the doors of our evolution. It restores our ability to find what we've lost, to see the missing piece. In this approach, we achieve healing when we're able to embrace the illness and its message. We can act from a place of acceptance. We can move toward health. To curse, to fight or to battle the problem actually empowers it as an enemy and increases its resources. The emotional condition of being in permanent conflict fosters an unfavorable biochemical state.

By the way, this calls to mind the many programs that exist to fight various diseases, especially the catastrophic ones. This includes foundations, groups, individual programs and massive public campaigns. I don't share their perspective on the so-called *fight*, but of course I still welcome them as viable options that are working to help people.

Fortunately, I also see that we're moving forward, albeit still with baby steps. More and more people are changing their perspective. They're changing how they see and react to what happens to them. The work I do and to which I've dedicated my life is making gains.

I'm increasingly encouraged to see more people interested in working internally, taking charge of themselves, more able to be honest with themselves and to address their illnesses and crises in a more holistic and open way. It takes a large dose of heartfelt sincerity to find and then air out our many shadows. They can be hard to get to and harder still to admit. But that sincerity of the heart allows us to see an opportunity where before we only saw pain or punishment. There's no room there for a fight.

Every illness is sacred, because it refers us to ourselves. It invites us to understand why we've created it and to look at the inner truth we've avoided. It gives us a map we didn't have. In this way, it becomes an inseparable pairing of health and disease: polarities with a common essence. By embracing one, we embrace the other. Our capacity to take charge of our health invites a journey and every journey has a starting point, which is different for each traveler. But it always involves an awareness of the need for change. In this case, the inception of the journey requires a connection with that best of guides, the most wonderful, ancient model of what we now call a GPS: the heart. At the end of the day, if we let ourselves be led, our heart guides us. And there will always be a luminous ending.

ACTIONS FOR A R.E.A.L. LIFE

Close your eyes and look at your ailment, whatever is happening to you, whether physical, mental or emotional. Connect with it from your heart.

Visualize it in front of you and say to it, "Now I see you with new eyes. Please reveal to me your mission in me; let me know what you want to show me. Now I say, yes, thank you, and I trust in the greater good you bring me."

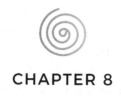

CHAPTER 8

THE R.E.A.L. THERAPEUTIC MODEL

"With a serene mind and an open heart, all roads open."
— ANONYMOUS

Gradually, through the experience of my practice, I designed my own model of accompaniment. I arrived at this method through my training, many years of practice, giving talks and workshops, and my own healing. It's the foundation of the therapeutic work I follow and it's also become my system for individuals. I've named it R.E.A.L., which is an acronym:

Resources that
Empower you
for **A**uthenticity
and self-**L**oyalty

I'm presenting my model here in a formal, organized way for the first time. It's not a closed or rigid model. I think of it more as a general guide for dealing either as a practitioner with cases or with oneself. It's like a connecting thread, like the string that joins the pearls and allows a group of separate, little jewels to become one beautiful necklace.

After I'd begun my practice, I studied in Spain for a master's degree in biological medicine, which is how they used to refer to integrative medicine. This helped me to organize various medical disciplines I'd studied in medical school in a fragmented way. I began to see things differently, with greater therapeutic maturity. I created a rhythm and a certain methodology to bring to my cases. I was more focused at the time on treating the physical but I discovered that, depending on the timeline of the patient's illness or the stage in which they arrived, I could adapt this new way of working.

I applied it to people suffering from various physical ailments, especially chronic and degenerative diseases (including many cases of cancer) with complex situations and vital organs compromised. Over time I was able to verify that if we initiated the treatment process with a detoxification, with nutritive changes and purifying treatments, it made a difference. It definitely made the body more receptive to everything else. Regardless of whether the treatment was conventional, integrative or a combination of both, the body was more available and responded much better. In many cases, when we began this way, I saw changes at the beginning of the process.

Gradually, while incorporating new therapeutic approaches, like the transformational, psychological and systemic, I began to wonder how I could apply these steps to other spheres of being. Thankfully, I was able to adapt the physical model to the emotional and found that, because it's based on general principles of life, it works in much the same way.

I came to view it as a kind of alchemy, which the ancients viewed as a science and a way to turn base metals into gold. But alchemy was also a metaphor for the process of human transformation and that's what this model can do. It facilitates changes inside you in the physical, mental, emotional, vital and spiritual planes, resulting in a healthier, proactive and happier life. It's something you can generate from a conscious commitment to yourself and your healing process.

The R.E.A.L. method suggests the action of preventing, maintaining, transforming, regenerating and revitalizing all the layers or aspects of being. The first step is to become aware of what we are, when we are, how we function and what part of us can improve. Then we can take advantage of that natural capacity that we've been given to repair and restore ourselves. It doesn't involve becoming someone different. It's about bringing forth a better version of ourselves.

This model may be unattractive to those who are looking for the easy and quick, although that doesn't mean it can't be both. But what I'm proposing is a path, a process toward transformation and the adoption of a way of thinking and living. I mean living from a connection with love, with the luminous, which results in in a commitment to yourself. That commitment is what allows you to deepen and make real change, because it involves constant observation and self-responsibility. In this model, at those points on the journey where a person seeks help, the therapist and patient form a team. They give feedback to each other and each fulfills their role.

The human being is always in motion and that flow is circular. We're exposed to challenges, new experiences and, if you will, new "toxins." We enter into cycles where we either go forward or stagnate. This is why the R.E.A.L. model suggests a periodic review on a case-by-case basis, like the maintenance we give equipment (changing the oil and filters in our car, defragging our computer, updating programs and the like). I sometimes describe this movement as an ascending spiral. Thanks to our experience and new awareness, we come back around to see the same things from higher level of understanding.

As I've said, the model isn't rigid and can't be because everyone is unique, with a particular history and different physical, emotional and mental characteristics. Everyone has a particular way of looking at life and what happens to them. We're not simply working with labels, diseases or diagnoses, although we take them into account. We work with the whole person, with what happens to them and how they respond. Therefore the work is individualized and different options are proposed. It's like getting a tailored suit as opposed to a standard size.

During the process, the reaction of the patient speaks to us and gives us guidelines. Understanding what the body says and how the emotions respond is what allows us to see the next step and to make necessary adjustments on the fly. Each person's history is a world of possibilities. Consequently, this way of working requires creativity from both sides. It's ultimately more of an art: the art of healing.

Experience has taught me that the steps of this approach work when a person truly wants to investigate. They facilitate relief. That said, I don't mean to invalidate the many patients who improve their symptoms without trying an approach which investigates the background of their problems. A patient can be physically cured and the holistic healing process I'm describing doesn't necessarily have to occur. Everything can remain at the level of finding a physical cure and that's also perfectly valid.

R.E.A.L. takes into account that human beings have a special wisdom in their design, with their own mechanisms of control. In addition, they have intelligent information and feedback systems to self-regulate, naturally and spontaneously. All of this happens at the cellular level, in the tissues and also at corresponding mental and emotional levels. These are mechanisms of reactivation, renewal, balance, adaptation and elimination.

But over time there's a normal deterioration of these mechanisms as well as various life changes and impacting events. They begin to work less efficiently. On the physical level, this means cell deterioration and changes in the inner environment or structure. On the emotional level, we create protective shells and survival mechanisms. These mechanisms help us to get where we are but they become what prevent us from regaining our strength, reconnecting with the center and recovering our equilibrium. This sustained inefficiency, which can start at any age in a variety of ways, can become a physiological or systemic stress to our vital organs that eventually affects the body's responsiveness and produces disease.

The events most frequently identified as causing damage to the system are physical, mental or emotional stress, inadequate nutrition, environmental contamination (of various kinds), lack of rest, lack of physical activity, unresolved conflicts and physical or mental trauma. These are mostly the result of one's lifestyle and emotional management.

Ideally, we would all be able to control the variables on which our health depends. It would also be ideal if we raised our emotional intelligence so we could understand our mechanisms of emotional reaction. Unfortunately, the concept of prevention in orthodox medicine is still very limited and a long way from this inclusive, comprehensive approach.

For obvious reasons, given how we live today, human beings tend to become unbalanced at an earlier and earlier age. This causes dysfunction. And when dysfunction begins (whether organic or emotional), or when a process of physical degeneration begins, we should act.

It bears repeating that this kind of approach is useful for any health issue, but especially in the treatment of chronic (long-term, slow-developing) illnesses and degenerative diseases. The idea is to stimulate the body to self-reregulate and collaborate from its own innate, curative resources. An integrative approach favors the least invasive treatments necessary to restore and maintain life and raise it to the best possible level of quality. But it also includes a variety of therapeutic approaches, including those of mainstream medicine. Still, given whatever the actual state of deterioration allows, the bias is toward the most natural treatment possible, with a minimum of drugs and managing the condition with more energetic and humanistic methods.

The R.E.A.L. method proposes five fundamental actions, which I call the five Rs:

**REVIEW
REMOVE
REPAIR
REVITALIZE
RESIGNIFY**

Together, these are the five fundamental pillars of a method for reversing the degenerative conditions of deep emotional stagnation, repetitive behaviors and chronic, toxic thoughts that are obstacles to the work of prevention.

The phases of R.E.A.L. aren't linear or rigid. It's a guide that can be adapted to individuals at a particular point in time. When we're in tune with life, we continuously make leaps of consciousness and new connections. We receive internal revelations and understand more about ourselves. When we're in *R.E.A.L. mode* everything is incorporated and much of what previously happened makes new sense. The veils are torn away and new lights appear before our eyes. Our path becomes a spiral in permanent motion.

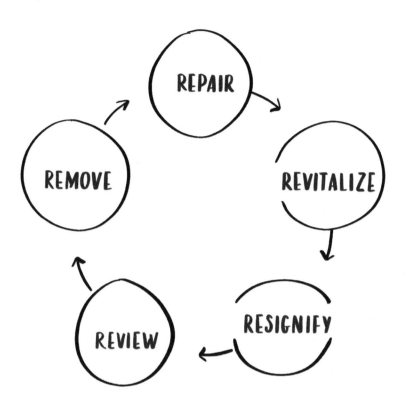

PART II

REVIEW

CONNECT WITH YOURSELF.

SOCRATES

CHAPTER 9

REVIEW:
YOUR HISTORY IS
YOU

*"The better you know yourself,
the better equipped you'll be for life."*

— GREGG BRADEN

This is the starting point. It's the great first step that directs us inward to understand who we are, what happened in the past and what's happening now. This allows us to place ourselves in a context, an actuality which we can then transcend. Whether we have a sickness or not, whether we're going through a crisis or not, we all need to know ourselves, to be in touch with ourselves and our inner truth. *Review* is the first resource that guides us toward our goals and empowers us to live with open eyes.

As you *Review* you begin to understand the process; what happened before and what led you to ask questions or seek help. It's about your life story, including your conscious reason for consultation and when and where the impulse started. It's not always a simple process. It involves patience, being attentive and actively listening. To go back to your beginning and to start a review from your very origin can bring all sorts of things to light. These can include physical or emotional impacts, forgotten facts, things that were said or unconscious decisions that changed your way of thinking and living, though at the time you may not have understood them. Now suddenly they begin to make sense, which already initiates healing, as something starts to be released. Only by shining the light of awareness can we see things that have been hidden in shadows. This is how the process becomes viable.

There's a story behind every human being and an integrative approach takes this into account. I'm dividing the inquiry into parts, but I only do so to make it easier to explain. Because actually the story is one. Everything that occurs at any level is part of the whole and contributes to its interconnectedness and the underlying reality we want to reveal.

When a patient sits before me, I consider that something specific moved them to seek help and it's often more urgent to focus initially on that, because of a real or apparent need. I say apparent, because sometimes there's a conscious reason for the consultation which is actually just the excuse to come. A whole avenue of discovery can follow, far beyond what motivated the person to ask for help.

We need a starting point and that's either the physical history, the emotional history or the family system, because ultimately all are interwoven and all relate to the issue at hand, even if this isn't always apparent.

In the words of Dr. Pablo Rubén Koval, one of my professors of neural therapy, "The life history is a way to know the process that this particular patient went through to develop the health problems for which they've come to consult. It's the story of the irritations and the reactions of their nervous system, both physically and emotionally, as well as the changes these alterations have caused in their relationship with the totality of their environment."[4]

When I studied neural therapy, my skills of observation and inquiry began to improve. It sharpened my perception of energy (which was already part of my work) and also my awareness of its obstructions. That's when I started to notice other potential interferences with health, to better understand the effects and blockages that arise from the physical or emotional history and affect the whole.

Once again, I realized that it's not just a matter of understanding the type of impacting event, but understanding the individual who is being impacted and their state when it happens.

Everyone processes experiences differently. That's why many physical reactions – such as post-surgery – aren't necessarily an indication that the procedure was done poorly. They're often the result of how that particular body processes new information. The body is integrating these new events with historical ones. The therapeutic approach is complex and unique to each individual.

Neural therapy, in particular, is a modality that's allowed me to look more clearly at the complexity of the communication of body parts and even the body's records. It's an injectable therapy, applied to specific parts of the body. It may be hard to believe that apparently disconnected physical parts communicate with each other, but they do.

I've had many experiences of this type. For example, I've injected the area that corresponded to an impacted tooth, a third molar, and instantly relieved a pain in the patient's knee. On another occasion, having intervened with neural therapy into a pelvic surgical wound, the patient went through a catharsis of reliving several failed pregnancies which she had never fully mourned. Even more surprisingly, I once treated the oral cavity and tonsillar poles of a patient, who then had a spontaneous regression to infancy. A few months after birth he'd been diagnosed with oral cancer and the injection I gave him brought up the traumatic experience.

These cases are among many I've encountered that demonstrate how if the body is *touched* in a particular way it can connect with related physical or emotional memories.

These cases also demonstrate the significance of those original events, and most importantly, the fact that there's no separation of our many parts. Finally, they illustrate something I emphasize throughout this book: everything is recorded in the body, even events that aren't particularly dramatic. Our entire history is there and biography definitely becomes biology. So making a comprehensive history of significant events, diseases and painful situations in one's life (as chronologically accurate as is possible) is an important part of what helps us decide where and how to approach treatment.

The Physical-Energetic

The *Review* is much like the usual medical history, in which you start by looking at whether the person is a woman or a man, their age, where they're from and so on, plus the reason for the consultation. The current situation is identified and the exam proceeds to the organs and systems.

This step in the exam is about getting to know the person's body, how it reacts, its strengths and weaknesses, and in what condition it arrived. What's the issue and who is the person before me? Does this body have the capacity to respond, to reverse processes? What's the level of preservation or deterioration? How did the issue develop and what's the lifestyle of this person?

This includes a conventional diagnosis, if there is one: the symptoms and the history of the condition itself, when and how it began, if it's associated with another event, how it has evolved and if it's associated with another event. Is there a pre-existing condition? What were the significant impacts such as falls, fractures, surgeries, dental extractions, implants, teeth in poor condition and infections? And what was the timeline of each of these conditions? The chronology is important. In short, the goal is to have as broad a picture as possible of the person's story.

This is also true of the analytics, including whatever tests results the patient already has or those we request. There's also the possibility of making referrals if we feel the need for a specialist's expertise.

Then, in addition to the conventional check-up and general physical exam, we add an energetic check-up (pulse, face, tongue, body language, kinesiology, iridology, the analysis of living blood, and so on).

In energy medicine

In addition to many methods geared to prevention, there are also excellent means for diagnosis. This is the case with pulses as well as diagnosis by the face in TCM. Certain signals can be read that indicate a problem which is developing but not yet otherwise symptomatic. The senses are also our allies because we can diagnosis by listening, looking, palpating or smelling.

Clearly, a medical visit like this takes more time than many doctors ever take in an initial visit. Listening and observation require dedication and enough time to be able to make a thorough review. This is what allows for truly individualized treatment.

The emotional aspect

In addition to the personal history after birth, a complete *Review* includes knowing what happened in childhood from the beginning of the mother's pregnancy. That means knowing what happened during this gestation period and even before, if the mother had any illness, physical or emotional threats, what her pregnancy was like, as well as the delivery and the beginning of life.

About 15 years ago, a little book fell into my hands that related different personality types to the nature of a person's birth. At the time I didn't really question whether it was based on serious research or not, it just made a lot of sense to me. I looked at how I was born and the births of others around me and I saw interesting connections. The book listed different personality traits for people whose birth was cephalic (headfirst) or breech (feet or buttocks first) or a twin birth or a C-section, as well as if the birth was fast or slow and so on. Since it really caught my attention, I continued to make these kinds of observations. And, in most of the cases I investigated, I found a correlation. This made even more sense to me after I became familiar with therapies such as clinical psychosomatic, bio-decoding and what has been called The Sense Project.

As therapists, when we know more about these earliest stages, it's much easier to find explanations for the cases we encounter. I've always believed that nothing is random and everything happens according to interconnecting laws. Often we don't know these laws or don't have all the conscious information about what's happened. Or sometimes we just don't make the associations. But it's quite clear that everything in a person's story is relevant, from the moment of conception to the manner of the birth, from lactation and the bond with the mother through the first years of life. These things all shed light on subsequent repetitions and manifestations in our lives that sometimes lack an apparent physical explanation.

We can check how the emotional base was formed at each stage of growth – oral, anal and so on – all the way up to the chronological age when the person comes for consultation. The first seven years are fundamental to understanding how we react, our emotional wounds and our ongoing defense mechanisms, as well as our inner arguments, edicts or toxic phrases lodged in the unconscious. These things determine a great deal of our behavior, including how we relate, respond and react.

Going back to the moment of your conception, have you wondered or do you have information about the couple that

gave life to you? How was their union? What were the circumstances between them at the time, their environment
and their reality? What were your parents like as individuals? Are you the product of a reconciliation, or were your
parents in conflict? Was the sexual act violent? Were you a
surprise? Were they hoping you would be a different gen-
der? How were their finances? The number of children in
the family and their order is also very important. Even if
siblings are born to the same parents, they come at different moments in the family history and the different circumstances change everything. This is why it's said that each
child has a different father and mother, even when the parents are biologically the same. Everything can yield information. One can also consider what was happening at the
time on a community level, nationally or globally. Was it a
time of peace, of war, of tyranny?

This is about becoming a historian of your own life, so
you can begin or resume your healing from the beginning,
from the origin of this life's journey.

The familial aspect

You were born into the middle of a story already in motion.
In the midst of that, even the name you were given is not
casual. It's a continuation of that story. History is alive and
full of beliefs. It has dramas, countless events, truths that
have been told and truths that have been hidden. This history is part of all that happens to us in life.

Our story doesn't begin with our birth, though most
people record it that way. In fact, it doesn't even begin
with our gestation or even our conception. Our life is connected to that of our parents, to what happened to them and
what they inherited from those who preceded them. We're
part of the story of our ancestors. This is why it's important to know family history, at least the recent history, by
which I mean the three generations that precede you. In

the transgenerational approach we talk about those seven couples that most influence you and how they are a key to a great deal of useful information for self-knowledge. Your family tree holds many keys.

Sometimes things happen to us that are more linked to unresolved issues from previous generations than to present-day issues or our own progress. These are like *echoes of the past,* which is the title of a book by Carola Castillo, with whom I studied family constellations.[5] The systemic approach contends that we inherit an important story from our ancestors, and when we speak of ancestors, we don't just mean distant relatives from many years ago. Ancestry starts with our mom and dad.

In recent studies, it's been discovered how traumas also alter genes and that we can inherit those genetic mutations from our parents. Intergenerational trauma is thus not only passed through sociocultural environments, but also through DNA. This is a fascinating world where everything fits together.

There are various studies along these lines. Belgian researcher Natalie Zammatteo has written about a direct impact on the DNA for three generations.[6] There's a study by a team from Mount Sinai Hospital in New York with Holocaust survivors and their children who were born after World War II. The study, found that these Jewish survivors and their children had lower levels of cortisol than people who lived outside of Europe during the war.[7] Cortisol is a hormone produced by the adrenal glands above the kidneys. Low cortisol may cause symptoms of depression, tiredness, or weakness and may also be indicative of other diseases.

There's also the research of Dr. Amy Bombay, professor of psychiatry at Dalhousie University in Halifax, Canada, who has studied the impact of trauma and its repercussions across generations. Dr. Bombay is of Anishinaabe origin (an indigenous North American people) and her study was motivated by seeing the after-effects in her own family of grandfathers and uncles having been forced to attend residential schools for indigenous youths.

The purpose of these state-run institutions was to "civilize" indigenous youths by forcibly taking them from their families and stripping them of their culture and language. Many were also abused. In 2015, the landmark Canadian Truth and Reconciliation report called the policy "cultural genocide."

Dr. Bombay found that those who had a parent or grandparent who attended one of these schools were at greater risk for psychological disorders, suicidal ideation and suicide attempts. This was true of adults and young people.[8]

These kinds of tendencies can be transmitted through psychological and social pathways as well as genetically, but there's mounting evidence of epigenetic pathways involved in trauma transmission. Populations that have suffered collective, historical traumas have now been studied around the world and there's consistency in the results.

In any case, we now know that both experiences and the environment can activate or deactivate genes so that the function of these genes changes. These changes occur in the germinal line – that is, in the egg or sperm – and are transmitted generationally.

It follows that these transmissions of ancestral information also play an important role in our quest for healing and reconciliation. To learn why one's grandparents did something that was later repeated by one's parents can help us to learn how to change the pattern. It can help us heal for ourselves and for other generations.

Scientific evidence that intergenerational trauma can be transmitted biologically will eventually lead to greater access to treatment for people all over the world who live with the effects of ancient tragedies engraved in the depths of their cells. Healing our history opens our lives to hope.

To close this topic, I want to mention positive lineage, so as not to dwell only in the drama of the negative and difficult patterns. Much of your life's richness, your skills and gifts, come from your ancestral group, from the legacy of the experiences of those who were part of your clan and who established your life's *programmation*. There's much to heal, but you've also been given many treasures.

Knowing your story gives you a context. It grounds you and it gives meaning to much of what happens to you. From there, the invitation is to consciously take steps that allow you to reconcile with your history and then redirect your story down your own path. To be loyal to yourself. I hope the adventure of life becomes a great opportunity for you, to live what's yours to live by acknowledging your full history.

I'll include below a few practices that have helped me and many of my patients to tune in to their own history.

ACTIONS FOR A R.E.A.L. LIFE

Collect information about what was happening in your country on the day you were born, as well as the world situation at the time. Learn about your parents' family situation during your time in utero and at your birth.

Write down relevant information from when your mother was pregnant with you, and important data from your birth. Write down significant facts from your childhood and adolescence. Includes moves, important events, travel . . .

In chronological order, write down your medical history: diseases you've had, surgeries, etc. Identify how you experienced each and consider what may have changed from them.

Collect your medical records. Organize the relevant information so you can share it with any professionals you consult.

Make your family / health tree. Include at least three generations. Note their names with dates of birth and death, economic conditions, professions, misfortunes and other relevant facts. Start with whatever information you have.

Close your eyes and think about how you came into the world. Imagine your parents behind you, your grandparents and your great grandparents and then envision the antecedent generations leading further and further back as far as you can imagine. See yourself as a result of these many events. Take a deep breath and accept all that's happened. Only then can you be here and be who you are. Ask permission from your heart to change and give thanks. Reconciling with history is the first step.

Integrate into your life this phrase: "I feel that life rewarded me and gave me the best possible history, with the best possible circumstances to place me where I am today, showing me the perfect keys to return to the R.E.A.L. in me and manifest the best version of myself."

CHAPTER 10

THE SYSTEMIC APPROACH TO PHYSICAL HEALTH

*"Your family tree has many of the keys you need
to expand your consciousness and to heal your body."*

— RAQUELINA LUNA

The knowledge of our ancestry gives us another perspective. It brings another reality into the light. This approach allows us to look at the origin of a disease at an alternate, complementary level, linked to the family of origin.

Dr. Stephan Hausner, one of the pioneers of constellation work in the field of health, has written, "It's not possible to apply holistic medicine without including the family or the relevant social environment of the patient."[9]

Let's be clear that the physical treatment of an illness isn't part of the discussion in this chapter, but it is essential. The systemic contribution doesn't replace necessary forms of intervention, be they medical, psychological or other. Nor am I suggesting that these concepts replace quality of life and a healthy lifestyle. Quite the contrary.

But everything that happens can also be seen from a systemic point of view. It's another way to view any ongoing health condition (chronic symptoms, acquired or inherited diseases, congenital diseases, etc.) or any emotional, family or relationship situation that's frequently repeated. Because we can often relate these to family events and information, this approach becomes an excellent complement to medical or psychological treatments. Another reality emerges as part of the story and the healing process is triggered by new understanding.

In recent years, I've enriched my clinical work with the inclusion of a transgenerational perspective. Through this approach I've begun to observe an illness, its context and its systemic impact in the family. Part of the job is to be able to decipher – with a patient who's open to this approach – the hidden meaning, undisclosed by the symptom but obstructing the process of change. The idea is to arrive at an understanding of the transgenerational and sometimes psycho-genealogical family framework, to help see the loyalties and deep bonds where the illness is rooted. It's beautiful to look at a family or a genogram (a pictorial display of a person's family relationships and medical history), to see the lights and shadows of the family unconscious and integrate them into the personal work.

In the process of treating others, I've also learned to accept and respect when they don't believe something like this can help them or don't feel the need to investigate. They simply want relief from a symptom. I've also learned to respect the person who's deeply tied to a particular loyalty and finds it too easy to stay in their pattern and too hard to take decisive steps. Staying loyal, staying sick, has its benefits for them. The status quo is okay as it is.

But when a patient is open and ready, there's a movement in which they can be guided more easily to health and toward life. This movement simultaneously generates a more conscious experience of the illness. This internal commitment leads to healing. In many cases, it causes the symptoms to disappear. In others, if the body still has the capacity to respond, it can actually cure the disease. As Bert Hellinger has said, "A healing movement is generated and by revealing the hidden dynamic, the secret happiness of the illness loses its meaning, channeling it toward life and health."[10]

In a systemic approach, diseases are seen as coming via hidden dynamics in the family, which are often a "transgression of order." The disease comes to compensate in some way for an imbalance in the system. This notion comes from Hellinger, who identified three fundamental elements in every family system: hierarchy, belonging and balance. The illness of an individual is an attempt to restore order, an unconscious, loving act of the sick person to their family. Obviously, a blind love. Often the disease represents a rejected or excluded family member who has been denied the right to belong in the family, which is the system. The illness comes as an invisible loyalty or blind love to fulfill what's missing in the system. The disease or imbalance "waves a flag" to draw our attention. It appears in a form we can see and so restore a balance. When we can include those who were excluded and restore them to a place of love and acceptance in the family, we give new momentum to the movement of healing. The sickness becomes a guide for the restoration of order: the order of love. That's how the system heals, which is to say, the family heals.

This "transgression of order" as a cause of illness has parallels in other healing traditions. Take for example the system of the five phases or five mutable kingdoms in TCM. Here we find the same essential conclusions: illness is viewed as a matter of order.

Perhaps it's important to remember that the disease appears in the family not because its members are bad people, but because within and through the family they act out destinies that involve, influence and affect all its members.

There are various examples of unconscious phrases connected with the family system that contribute to generating illness or even death. For example, sometimes a child's loving *antennae* perceive that their father or mother wants to die or is mortally ill and, internally and unconsciously, says, "I'll do it in your place." There's a death-wish behind many addictions.

In cases like I mentioned above, where an individual has been excluded, another family member's internal voice might say, "I will follow you into exile," or "I'm replacing you." In chronic depression, one parent has often been excluded.

In some cases, the family's hidden dynamic is that the mother (or father) tells the child, "Everything that comes from your father (or mother) and his family is worthless. You should only take after me." This denies the child access to that parent.

When a person has issues of order with their parents and is in a position of too much dominance, we may find the unconscious phrase, "I'm stronger and I can do more than you."

When there's a very sick person in the family system, the phrase might be, "I'll follow you in sickness," "I'll go in your place," or "Me instead of you."

Behind incidences of cancer in women, constellations have often revealed pending issues with the mother such as rejection, or superiority over her, or a sense of blame. In some cases, they're generational. This is most commonly seen in cancers linked to female organs.

Physical health in general is usually related to the mother or is linked to the maternal pathway. Mental health is more related to the paternal line or the presence of the father.

When there are serious illnesses that are deeply painful for the individual and the entire family, a minimum of three generations can be impacted. These kinds of tragic events may even have happened before, several generations back. They repeat because there's an unconscious transgenerational passage not only of a genetic tendency, but also of values, emotions, experiences, mandates and loyalties.

All these observations arise from the therapeutic work of many researchers, studying diseases and their entanglements from a systemic point of view. As Stephan Hausner has said, "Whole health in its totality can only be felt by one who has taken in his heart all those to whom he belongs, who can look in the eyes of each one to whom he belongs and say "I accept it from you . . . and I keep it as something special."[11] When we have taken into our hearts both the easy and difficult, we attune ourselves to what we need.

Brigitte Champetier has described illness as a movement of the spirit which opens to us a complete process of reconciliation. The mission of health, she writes, is to reconcile ourselves with life, with the mother, with others and with ourselves. Through a powerful process of healing and growth, a sick person can heal a disorder for the whole system.[12] In this way, the family system can lose its rigidity and regain coherence at a new level of consciousness, allowing all of its members a greater autonomy and more life.

THE YES

Liberation and movement begin with a *yes*, which is an assent. When the person affirms all that they are, they set out toward resolution. First they take to heart the history that's happened without wanting to change it. Then they accept their situation as it is. This is the key to an adult understanding. With that *yes*, the sense of blame is released. A calm descends and the person can reconnect with life and take charge of what is theirs.

In other words, saying *yes* (which goes far beyond mere acceptance) means we stop denying, ignoring or wanting to change what simply was or is. Once we embrace that full reality without judging it or trying to dress it up or change it, we can start the movement of healing.

ACTIONS FOR A R.E.A.L. LIFE

Close your eyes for a moment and think about what's happening to you, what you haven't been able to fix, change, move or heal. No matter what kind of issue it is, bring it to consciousness. Envision your history behind you, represented by previous generations, starting with your parents. Draw strength from them and feel their support until from the bottom of your heart comes a yes!

Stay there until you feel it. You can repeat this yes as many times as you need until you feel the inner movement of total acceptance, tranquility and true assent.

CHAPTER 11

INTEGRATING MIND, BODY AND EMOTIONS

"Until the unconscious becomes conscious, the unconscious will continue to lead your life and you will call it destiny."

— CARL GUSTAV JUNG

Behind every damaged organ or physical pain, there's a disturbance at the emotional and/or mental level. I arrived at his comprehensive view of the human being through the study of TCM. Since then, through diverse currents of study and decades of practice, I've dug ever deeper into this reality.

It's good when a concerned patient vents their feelings or voices regrets. It's always beneficial to talk about what we're going through, especially with a good listener. But it's rare that a patient is awake or even open to the understanding that whatever particular physical concerns they have are literally linked to what's happening at other levels. Although it's also fair to say that this has changed a bit from when I first began my practice.

Psychosomatic is the term for an emotional or mental counterpart to a physical process. And though it's often accurate, the word has a terrible reputation. The WHO acknowledges that over 75% of illnesses are just that: a physical condition caused by an emotional or mental factor. Still, the word is rarely well received. Many people feel insulted. They interpret it to mean that their disease is imaginary or invented and that they're mentally disturbed. This partly provokes a resistance to seeing beyond the physical to the truth. It's completely understandable though, given how the subject is often addressed by professionals.

I partly attribute these attitudes to how little time is devoted to training in this aspect, both in medical school and in our own lives. In general, doctors are simply not prepared to approach matters of health from this perspective. Usually, the only time a psychosomatic cause is considered is when all else fails, when a patient doesn't improve by any method and the doctor can't find any obvious physical cause. The conclusion then is that the patient "has nothing" and their condition is "mental." I'm speaking about what I experienced in my own medical training and what I've seen with very few exceptions in 26 years of professional practice.

When I began to study TCM, I learned about *qi (chi)* or vital energy and how it stagnates when we have unresolved situations or emotional wounds from the past. If that energy is stagnant or latent for long periods, it accumulates and quietly begins to cause damage to the organs. Then physical or emotional consequences often end up triggering some symptom or disease.

More recently, many innovative ideas have emerged in the therapeutic world, some inspired by ancient traditional medicines and others based on personal experiences and enriched by new research. But these ideas are not completely new to science.

In the 1940s, psychologist Robert Ader and immunologist Nicholas Cohen, both researchers, opened a new paradigm for the scientific community with the discovery of the interaction between the nervous system and the immune system. Their work was later named psycho-neuro-immuno-endocrinology, though every bodily system could actually be included in this name, which would make it even longer. In any case, this name encompasses the connections of the mind to every part of our body.

Since then, neurosciences have been gradually providing many answers about the intercellular communication of immunology and genetics. There's increasing evidence that there's no division between the mind and body because of the interconnectedness of the brain, the nervous system and the endocrine and immune systems.

The biopsychosocial model is another way of conceptualizing medical reality and was first proposed in 1977 by George Engel. I first heard about it in medical school. Engel's proposal proceeds from the idea that the human being is intrinsically composed of biological, psychological and social factors and therefore a person's behavior and lifestyle can benefit or impair their health. Any stressful situation that disrupts one of the systems of human functioning affects the other systems via multiple mind-body connections.[13]

Psychoneuroimmunology is another model I learned about in the late 1990's while delving into studies on stress. Around that time, I also began to venture into neural therapy. I'd already been working with TCM, but I was happy to encounter evidence of cutting-edge research that confirmed these things from yet another point of view.

Since then, I've encountered various other models: German new medicine, the psychosomatic clinic, biodecoding, bioneuroemotion, and more.

The German new medicine, developed by Dr. Ryke Geerd Hamer in the early 1980s, postulates that diseases, including cancer, are the result of changes in the biological program caused by an unexpected impact or shock that takes the person off-guard and triggers a survival program in what he calls the *mind-brain-organ.* Once the impact or event is resolved, the body returns to normal.[14]

For me, these recent modalities all reflect a return to the original, holistic concept of medical-philosophy. This return is inspiring new scientific research and relaunching the idea that we're an integrated whole. This is affirmed in an exciting way by quantum physics, which offers even broader explanations, demystifies many of these topics and validates such new approaches. I'll return to quantum physics in a later chapter.

Little by little, we're finding links to ancient traditions, to the theories of energy found in almost all the Eastern models and which were adopted in the West by Hippocrates, Galen and others. Maybe it's a dream, but I hope with all my heart that this understanding will eventually be incorporated into the mainstream medical system and that the predominant Western approach will be enriched by these valuable contributions.

Although some of these kinds of connections are clear and quickly visible to a trained observer, they're not always simple to understand clinically. The link to an emotional or mental origin is often obscure and can be complex. Thus, it's important to understand that human beings have a conscious part and an unconscious part. The conscious content is relatively easy to discern because it's what we observe. It's the obvious: reasoning and understanding. But the content of the unconscious has to be gradually deciphered. And for this, our ally par excellence is the body, the container of all experiences.

Returning for a moment to the conscious, I say that it's relatively easy to discern because our culture ignores conscious emotions. Nor do we get any education about them. Much of the time we don't even know what to call an emotion so we simply say, "I feel bad." Our emotions are often repressed or denied, evaded or rationalized, so they're not always obvious even when we're staring at them. And of course, we're all partly blinded and biased by beliefs, dogmas, internal defenses and the rest. The point is, emotional intelligence should be an important subject in our education. We invest little to no time in it and when we do it's introduced as intellectual or technical content. In the realm of the unconscious, we enhance our perspective on a situation when we observe its origin and its implications. We enhance it further by recognizing that everything that happens to us at any level happens to our body and this affects our well-being, our health and the way in which we relate to others. Each part of the body records the history of what's happened in our lives. The body keeps this history, which we mostly forget and which is full of sadness, joys, dramas, impacting events, achievements, failures, rejections, abandonment and a long list of other experiences. Alice Miller says, "The truth of our childhood is stored in the body."[15] This history is built into its formation, its strengths and weaknesses. All is registered and still present. Negative emotions from the past may have created problems or subtly caused deep damage that initially goes unnoticed. Illnesses that apparently have no physical reason can eventually arise from energetic blockages caused by these historical recordings.

Recordings or emotional imprints are unconsciously housed at different levels in the body, both in neural networks and in the muscles. According to neuroscientist Candace Pert, "The memories are not only stored in the brain, but also in the psychosomatic network that extends throughout the body, along the connections between the organs and up to the surface of our skin."[16] All of this reaffirms the importance of personal history, every aspect of which leaves a psycho-corporal footprint.

Given this connection of mind, body and emotions, one could say that all diseases are fundamentally psychosomatic. They all have an implication on another level and they're all affected by physiological changes that occur in response to certain thoughts, emotions or sensations. Ultimately everything is biological.

Illness then, is the result of how we think and feel. It's also the result of how our energy is modified by our attitude toward our circumstances and events. It's not only caused by what happens to us but also how we react to what happens to us. This is why similar events can register so differently in the different people. Some have coping mechanisms to modify their responses. These are resources they've adopted through learning and experience.

Our responses are largely conditioned by our unconscious association with events recorded in our emotional memory that either were or weren't released. Those that weren't released or processed are blocked and with some later event they can emerge from anonymity, often oversized.

By way of illustration, it's common to find cases where a grief was not fully expressed or processed and in the face of a later loss – though perhaps a much lesser grief – the reaction is greater and more difficult for the person to overcome. It may seem exaggerated but it's actually a response to the previous, unresolved grief that was buried and now both griefs combine. It's as if the recent grief uncovers the previous one. Adolfo Díaz says, "Emotional pain is like water; if you cover it, sooner or later it will find a way out."[17]

Let's consider those deeply buried, guarded emotions. Suppose we face a situation that theoretically shouldn't provoke distress but does? Or our reaction to something that happens is apparently exaggerated? Or we suddenly react in an unusual or unexpected way? We can respond by asking ourselves, "What's the past emotion that was blocked?" Or, "What might've been locked away, unacknowledged, in some deep place in me that's just been released by something relatively small?" Regardless of the emotion, if a visceral reaction surprises you or the intensity or duration of it doesn't correspond to what happened, or you're suddenly out of control, go to your history. Review what might've happened before, even back to whatever childhood wounds are there: inadequacies, devaluations, abandonment, rejections, violence, fears, betrayals or humiliations. No doubt you'll find something. In other words, observing our reactions can be an excellent way to find clues as to what's unresolved in our unconscious.

This brings us to the famous theme of the inner child, and the notion that all that happens in childhood remains as a record of stored memories which are present in our later, adult experiences. Voltaire expressed it poetically, "What reaches the heart is recorded in memory by fire." Most of us come from injured inner children who had to adapt or react by creating defenses and protective patterns which we unconsciously repeat until as adults, hopefully, we make them conscious. But many of these defense mechanisms need a little help in order to be deactivated. Until that happens, we continue as adults just like we did in childhood, in "survival mode."

Neuroscience has taken a path inspired by Sigmund Freud, the controversial father of psychoanalysis. Freud posited various ideas about the unconscious as a starting point and some have evolved considerably, especially in the analysis of human duality. Recent research in this field, along with convergent evidence from many scholars, is demonstrating ever more clearly that a large part of our mental activity is unconscious or automatic and that conscious activity is just the tip of the iceberg.

For example, Mark Solms, a neuropsychologist at the University of Cape Town, South Africa, reminds us that while the conscious mind is able to attend to six or seven things at once, our unconscious takes care of hundreds of simultaneous processes, from the vital organs, which are governed by the nervous system, to many of our daily decisions.[18]

In individual consultation, as well as in group talks and workshops, I often use the well-known iceberg metaphor to illustrate the contents of our consciousness. Looking at the iceberg, above the water's surface we see the tip. But this represents just 5-10% of the whole iceberg. That small percentage corresponds to the conscious mind. In other words, what we know, what we learn, what we realize and what we can rationally analyze and understand is a small percentage of our content. The base of the iceberg, which is covered by water and not visible from the surface, corresponds to the unconscious and represents 90-95% of our total content.

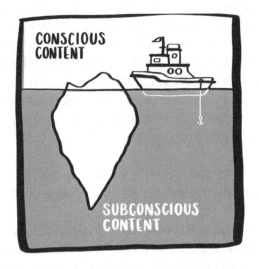

Somewhere in that unconscious 90-95% is the childhood story we don't remember. And the fact that we don't remember it is a mechanism of protection and survival. It includes the wounds of our inner child, the magical experiences, its healthy parts, fantasies, the repressed and expressed desires, the rejected and validated feelings, the emotions and impulses. This whole story affects the adult that we've become. But the unconscious is not just a trunk or sea-chest of memories and forgotten events. It's an internal world in which there are also unknown dynamic forces with programmed and adaptive responses. It's also linked to the family unconscious, the social collective and the evolutionary process. This is a topic that is as interesting as it is extensive. My goal here is to highlight the value and relevance of the unconscious – the protagonist of much of who we are – and to link it to health. If most of our content is stored in the unconscious, it's responsible for much more than we think, much more than just the rational and conscious. The unconscious directs us in far-reaching decisions such as our profession, the choice of our partners, where we live and so forth. It also directs us in our diseases.

Humans have a great capacity for adaptation, even to the point of not perceiving many of the repercussions of our experiences. There's a great disconnect of the body from our sensations and feelings. This is why we often don't even realize that what happens to us is linked to stagnant or trapped emotions in the body. We only know the result: physical discomfort, rigidity, lack of achievements in our pursuits, the repetition of painful events and on and on. We notice the effects. And in a culture whose concept of healing is based on suppressing the symptom or symptoms of an illness, much of this information is ignored.

At the psychic level, we acquire a series of habits that are also translated to the body without us noticing. The body is at the service of the unconscious and is the repository of anything not looked at, not expressed or not consciously processed.

We're also subjected to a generally high level of stress due to the demands of everyday life. This is also registered in our bodies, enough to cause them to shrink by the end of the day. Curiously, sometimes the level of tension in my body is such that at dusk I'm a few centimeters shorter than I was at dawn.

The continuous state of adrenaline which is now practically our norm also produces a sensory contraction and an ongoing state of alert so that the muscles are in constant tension. The body's ability to adapt helps keep us from constantly reacting to this tension, because the homeostatic mechanisms are functioning at their maximum. They try to compensate and keep us balanced. But this creates a virtually permanent stress on the organs that's also registered in the body and can eventually collapse the system and cause a permanent imbalance.

Continuous tension tends to cause us to lose body integration, including muscle tone. We lose the connection with our body memories, with our proprioceptive perception (awareness of the body in space) and our visceral sensation. We enter into mere survival mode and a kind of automatism. We'll go into this further in Chapter 29, which is an in-depth discussion of stress.

Sometimes we're surprised at the onset of a terrible, catastrophic disease and we wonder, "What happened? Why this?" The process of imbalance is long and silent and involves many factors, such as lifestyle, diet, rest and other physical habits. But it's worth highlighting the role played by those other, unconscious factors which are sometimes so intangible and misunderstood. They are equally powerful in causing biological changes and the triggering of what we call disease. They have a lot to do with why a person can get sick despite taking very good care of themselves.

This brings us back to the notion of the multidimensionality of human beings and the interdependence of our parts. Whatever happens can't be viewed reductively or as isolated. Spiritual progress is not enough, nor is emotional work, nor a good diet and proper care of the body. We need to act on all of these fronts. We are integral but multi-faceted beings and we need to travel diverse roads all the way to the point where they converge.

In this unity that we are, anything that benefits or harms one part affects another in a comparable way. We could say that the body and mind mirror each other. We could add that the parts of our bodies that don't work well reflect parts of our mind-emotions that also don't work well. The body becomes the sensor or monitor.

Once again, my proposal is that we work at all levels and use whatever information we can gather first from any of the parts to connect us to the rest. And very often the part that guides and *speaks* to us most is the body. It constantly gives us away. The underlying principle of psycho-corporal work is an understanding of all these *recordings* in our bodies and how we can release them.

Often, in addition to purely emotional processes, physical interventions are necessary. Some of the therapies that are directed at the body can help unblock that which is rooted to the body and doesn't emerge easily into consciousness. This is why psycho-corporal therapies can be so valuable in treatment. They can give us greater access to the interior of the person.

Energy therapies also play an important role in this regard, not only to improve physical or emotional ailments, but also to help things emerge and bring them to the conscious plane. Any psychological or mental program of treatment, be it psychotherapeutic, orthodox or humanist, is greatly enhanced by specialized work with the body. Of course, it may also be necessary to medicate, change the diet or apply other resources to balance the body.

By working, feeling and releasing each organ and muscle structure, you become aware, you free and heal yourself in the mental dimension which opens a path of expression for inner strength. It's often true that even just bringing a trauma to consciousness is enough to start the liberating movement.

CHAPTER 12

EMBRACING YOUR BODY

"The reason I have great discomfort is because I have a body. He who values the world as much as his body can be entrusted with the Empire. He who loves the world as much as his body can be entrusted with the Empire."

— TAO TE CHING

Unconsciously, the body is the repository of our guilt, compulsive needs, missing pieces, emotional holes and lack of recognition. It's the repository of all our wounds and shortcomings.

Lack of acknowledgement refers, once again, to all that we ignore, our lack of connection to self-love, often with great self-devaluation. This is where we encounter the quest for the *perfect body*. I'm struck by the increasing number of cosmetic surgeries, especially among women. This constant striving for the ideal, perfect physique moves me to reflect on how we actually value ourselves.

I'm not against looking better, nor am I against cosmetic surgery. I'm just calling attention to what may be hidden behind the often-anxious pursuit of such "adjustments." Looking good, maintaining your weight, being toned – these are all positive things. While accepting the fact that much of what I see in the mirror is not the same as it used to be, I also want to look good. And I confess that sometimes it hasn't been easy to see in myself the marks of time: new wrinkles, deeper lines of expression, loss of muscle tone, my skin less bright and smooth. Sometimes it's hard to compare new photos with old ones and to say in a loving way, "Yes, that's me too," and that's understandable. The body is a vehicle that allows you to relate, interact and communicate with the world around you and with your inner world. It's not all that you are. At the same time, without it you are not. In other words, the body alone is nothing but without it there's no expression of who you truly are. For me, it makes a lot of sense to understand that if what we are – our essence – requires the body, then it really is a kind of temple. It harbors the essential. Without it you cannot feel, without it you cannot think. Without it you cannot enter into connection with the sublime or exercise your spirituality. Spirituality starts with your body. The body makes possible everything that happens to us. It allows us to receive the impact of outside forces and it gives us our inner sensations. Through it we express what we are. In the words of Walt Whitman, "If anything is sacred, the human body is sacred."

This has often caused me to reflect on spirituality. It has led me to questions such as, "Is there true spirituality without connection to the body? Or without respecting it or without its recognition or care?" And, "How can I consider myself spiritual if I don't embrace my body? If I don't even understand its language? If I'm not in touch with what it tells me?" Nothing subtle, sublime, spiritual or inspiring, can happen without the body. Given that, my sense of spirituality begins with the body, with respect and a connection to that which gives me the possibility of transcendence, to that which makes it possible to commune with my essence. A lack of respect for the body implies a lack of care, mismanagement, abandonment and even abuse.

The body is also your great ally in the process of growth and identification with yourself. Its shape, its characteristics are not casual and respond to what you are. Besides, the senses reveal to you what happens. They show you the truth and are among your most valuable resources of self-knowledge. Listening to the body then, becomes a powerful tool of personal work.

As I've said, nothing that you experience escapes the body's records. Your cellular memory includes emotional, physical, mental and even transgenerational information, which conditions you in one way or another. It conditions your behavior, your reactions, your mannerisms, how you relate to people and events and how you handle stress and other challenges.

Luis Díaz compares the body to a computer. The holistic being is like the hard disk. The cellular memory as a whole is like the database of that disk and the countless, individual cellular memories are the files in the database. Everything that's ever happened to us, Díaz writes, is recorded in the cells of our body like digital files. "Stored in our cell memory are all the conscious and unconscious imprints of unproductive behaviors that don't allow us to feel happy and healthy enough to achieve our goals by awakening to our potential."[19]

Life is a dance of polarities and this is also true of what's recorded in our bodies. One polarity has been called the *positive emotional charge*, which creates a fluid energy field and healthy movement that helps you maintain a balance. This charge is related to a sense of security, trust, love, freedom, expression and inner peace. Conversely, there's a *negative emotional charge*, created by traumas and painful experiences that are poorly processed. This charge is responsible for the stagnation and blockages of vital energy, so it's largely responsible for the imbalances that eventually cause an illness. Once again, that's why, even with healthy lifestyle, it's still not enough when there are conscious or unconscious emotional burdens that haven't yet been released or properly channeled. Understanding this is fundamental for a medical approach and for everything concerning emotional intelligence. It's worth clarifying that an emotion is not an imbalance. Emotions are human, normal, necessary and inevitable. What makes them harmful is when they're not processed properly so they overwhelm us for too long or when they're ignored or repressed and buried in a state of latency, in an unconscious form. Faced with the loss of a loved one it's logical to be sad, to feel pain and even anger or rage. It's normal to pass through a process of emotional highs and lows for a period of time. But if these feelings aren't processed and sufficiently resolved, subsequent consequences can occur and they can end up being expressed as a symptom or an illness.

Dr. Ryke Geerd Hamer, the founder of the German new medicine, dedicated himself to demonstrating this dynamic of disease and emotional conflict after he and his wife experienced it first-hand. Their son was the victim of a shooting and died. This tragic loss, compounded by the complications and difficulties of the judicial investigation, deeply affected the Hamer couple. After four months, Dr. Hamer developed testicular cancer. His wife, Dr. Sigrid Hamer, suffered through several consecutive types of cancer and then died from a sudden heart attack. These events led to the birth of German new medicine.[20]

This and other similar schools of thought have been classifying symptoms and diseases and ascribing their emotional origins in a specific and detailed way. All of this knowledge and research has reinforced the understanding we inherited from TCM and other ancient traditions that linked the organs with the emotions.

Not all diseases occur as quickly as those described in the Hamer case. Many times an illness develops from emotional loads which are deeply buried and have already passed to an unconscious level, making it more difficult to link them to an emotional origin. This is why it helps us to review the detonator or trigger of the event, which leads us by the hand to the possible resolution.

We can walk through life without realizing that we're carrying a great burden of anger, anxiety, fear, guilt or resentment. Eckhart Tolle called this the "body of pain."[21] It feeds on emotionally painful energies and negative thoughts. In some people it becomes an addiction to unhappiness and drama. The "body of pain" can have an active phase and a dormant one. When dormant, it hides in the unconscious, as if inside us there's a sleeping volcano. The dormant period varies from person to person. Sometimes it can sleep for years until a particular event awakens it. As Marianne Costa says, "Everything we manage to hide ends up manifesting in our body."[22]

The body is the great talker and doesn't lie. It gives us away and shows us the truth, often in spite of ourselves. Our minds or our words may try to deceive, but not the body. In this way, our own structure provides us with the way to heal.

Many times, working with the body is the best way to set memories in motion and release blocked physical areas. Then one can complete the process with conscious work. Working with the body is also effective with children, since they can't always process emotional memories like adults. In general, regardless of what's involved and the ease or difficulty of integrating emotions into the circular gaze of the holistic approach, it's valuable and sometimes essential to work simultaneously on both the body and emotions to achieve a full resolution.

Focusing on the body also makes it easier to be more in touch with our vital center, the core where we experience life and the best of ourselves. It helps us to experience our own presence and intimacy. This is body intelligence,

partly. The great challenge is to be able to truly begin a relationship of dialogue with the body, where it becomes more prominent and we can receive its warnings through mindful, ongoing attention to our sensations and physical states.

Body intelligence connects us to the present moment. If we're more present in and through our bodies, more attentive to what happens, then we avoid much of the pain caused by escaping the present.

Escaping the present means being preoccupied, either with what's already happened and no longer exists or in the expectation of the future, which doesn't yet exist. Neither is real. The real, the truth, is here and now. Being caught up in the past or future is a distraction or a way to flee and it often keeps us suffering. That's what causes stress. The consciousness of the here and now leads us to what actually is and this can only be lived through the body. It's the present moment, the one when things happen.

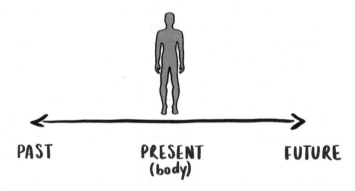

PAST   PRESENT   FUTURE
                    (body)

By now, we should be able to consider the body in a fresh and far more dimensional way. So when we talk about care, it's about going beyond the so-called culture of well-being and personal care, though obviously still taking those things into account: healthy food, rest, exercise, personal hygiene and a cleanly environment. But now we can also include listening to our body and having an awareness of its signals and warnings.

The goal is to connect more and more with the body, as much as possible. So the questions you might ask yourself are, "What can I do to really feel my body? How can I move more consciously?" Then start paying attention. Right now, continue reading but pay attention to your body and don't change anything. Notice your jaw. Notice your breathing. Is it complete? Is it shallow? What about your back or shoulders or chest? Are they held? Are they tense or are they relaxed? Notice the expression on your face (often a clue). Now start moving with this awareness. Do you realize how you move? Feel your body in all of its parts. How do they relate?

This is a small example of what you can start to do. The most important thing is to stay focused all the time. To keep coming back to yourself so that paying attention to your body gradually becomes a natural mechanism. Then in the midst of your daily life or when you get bad news or when someone contradicts you or says something you don't like, you can perceive more easily how your body reacts because you've trained yourself to pay attention.

We don't always hear what it says, but the body communicates constantly. It speaks through areas that contract, changes in our breathing, changes in temperature, sensations of opening, lightness or heaviness, postures, gestures and facial expressions. You get subtle messages when there's something that doesn't feel right to you. If you don't understand the signal, your body tends to express itself more obviously, perhaps as pain or more complex symptoms or intense negative emotions. This includes accidents, which are not casual and also have their significance.

At some point, everyone has felt their stomach tighten or their heart begin to race or they've broken out in a cold sweat from fear. When something suddenly makes you angry or ashamed you may have felt your jaw clench or your fists, a change in bodily sensations, temperature or even the color of your face. Emotional responses cause a cascade of chemical reactions in the body, stimulating some organ systems and inhibiting others. The reality is that these changes that occur from emotional reactions are what allow us to feel and identify them. Emotions and thoughts are not separate from the physical. It's normal and healthy to have such responses. Even emotions you don't like and consider negative, like fear and sadness, play a positive role in the right doses. Fear helps us remember caution, care and protection. It's one of our survival mechanisms. Sadness connects us with reflection, analysis and internalization. Anger connects us with energy to make things happen and overcome challenges. But again, when our reactions are severe, exaggerated and/or prolonged, depending on their duration and an individual's vulnerability, they create discomfort and can damage organs, making them more prone to disease.

Knowing yourself in a closer and more intimate way can help you develop self-awareness of your whole being. When you develop this awareness of your sensations and movement and bring it to a daily activity, it's as if you're a flashlight that shines on your own body. So it's not only a way to be more with yourself in everything you do, it's also a way to integrate what happens to you into your bodily structure, along with the accompanying emotions and thoughts. When you increase your ability to be present in yourself and know your own reactions, you know the areas of your body that get triggered. Then you can tell more easily when for example something sets off an old wound from your inner child. This helps you discover what things affect you more, as well as your true needs. It's a primary step toward growing in consciousness, reaffirming yourself and gradually changing what no longer works for you. Best of all, you can train yourself.

The body, as both a material vehicle and a repository of experiences, is an instrument of reconciliation and healing.

We have the perfect body to learn and grow. The more consciously we connect and reconcile with the body, the greater the possibility of moving toward personal power. The more we value, love and listen to our bodies, the more we integrate our own love. This includes honoring and accepting the changes that come with the passage of time.

Through bioenergetics, I came to understand much more of the relationship between these three elements: body, mind and energetic processes. Bioenergetic analysis is a therapeutic method that was first developed by Dr. Alexander Lowen from the work of Wilhelm Reich.[23] Reich was a disciple and contemporary of Freud who developed studies on the circulation of energy, the armor of the character and muscular armor.

Bioenergetic analysis, tells us that muscular stiffness from chronic tension can be caused by unresolved emotional conflicts. Usually, much of the physical tension that appears with acute stress disappears when the stress is relieved. Chronic tensions, however, persist after the initial stress is gone but, due to our natural process of physical adaptation, they're not always perceived. These chronic muscle stresses in turn disrupt emotional health by decreasing energy, restricting the play of natural and spontaneous muscular movements and limiting their self-expression. They become a circuit that feeds back: emotional stress produces chronic tension, which in turn decreases vital energy. This decrease in energy intensifies the emotional state. It takes work on the body to relieve that chronic tension and help recover vital energy and emotional well-being.

In addition to what a person thinks and expresses about themselves and their lives, bioenergetics takes into account the analysis of actual behaviors that either come into play or are avoided in sessions with the therapist. This includes emotions, attitudes and bodily movements and it requires attentive listening and observation of gestures and movements. The therapist must read the patient's body. This form of psychotherapy delves into what the body expresses and what it needs.

There are other resources that also work on the body, both structurally through manual therapies and which allow for recognition of the body's messages beyond the conventional approach to an injured organ or an already established disease. Among these resources I should mention the work of Adriana Schnake, a psychiatrist engaged in gestalt psychotherapy. One aspect of her work that I find both brilliant and relevant has been connecting gestalt work to physical diseases and symptoms. Taking off from Perl's *Gestalt Dialogues*, Dr. Schnake creates a technique for dialogue with different organs and bodily systems.[24] This technique provides another way to understand an organ or to bring to light repressed or buried information. And this information, combined with accessing the emotions, can bring change and can help the body to be open and available for that change.

Our natural self-healing capabilities are stimulated when we listen to the body's language without distorting it. As Schnake says, "Just as in any cell of the body is the total genetic structure of the individual, every organ contains the person's complete information."[25]

When you ignore the signs, you ignore the language of the body and distance yourself from its wisdom. The more attuned you are to the subtle messages of your nervous, digestive, and hormonal systems, the more and better you can adjust your behavior for greater well-being. It's important to pay attention to signals of satiety when we eat, to signals of our need to rest or to keep going, either physically or emotionally. When you're in harmony with the body and listen to it, you respect its wisdom.

Emotional intelligence truly rests on body intelligence, which is also key to the development of a healthy and empowered adult. If we understand what our body tells us and respect its signals, we're on the way to creating a relationship of love and well-being with ourselves.

I offer the following exercises below as a start to relating differently to yourself. They're intended to help you tune in and start designing your own plan for living with you. Enjoy this new love, your body.

Spirituality
BEGINS THROUGH
the body

ACTIONS FOR A R.E.A.L. LIFE

Begin body contact. Raise your hands gently to your heart. Talk to your body: "Dear body, I'm so sorry I haven't paid attention to you. I'm sorry I haven't listened except sometimes when I reach the limit. Thank you for sticking with me even if I don't pay attention to you." Just stay there a while, breathing.

Scan yourself in silence. No matter what position you're in right now, don't try to change it. Just pay systematic attention to the sensations in each part of you. Without judgement, simply pay attention to what's going on.

Check if there's one part more supported than another. Feel the temperature. Notice if there's any other sensation. In this way, review your whole body. If you do this regularly, you will notice in time that you're more alert with a greater presence in yourself.

Stay with this sense of scanning, be present in your body while you work, while you converse, while you exercise, when you arrive somewhere . . . make it a habit.

Embrace yourself, touch yourself affectionately. Apply oils and creams to your body and do so with a different awareness, massage yourself lovingly and with a sense of closeness and enjoy the new sensation.

CHAPTER 13

CORRESPONDENCES
IN THE BODY

"The heartbeat of our heart is our cathedral, our most sacred space. Those who cannot hear the heartbeat of their hearts suffered some aggression during their childhood."

— MARIANNE COSTA

A number of authors have dedicated themselves to the search for the meanings, correlations or correspondences of emotions and the body. These include Dr. Hamer, Louise Hay, Dr. Carbajal, Martell, Arrow, Corbera, and others. They've classified illnesses or body parts, trying to link them through those correspondences to the more subtle planes we've talked about, the emotional, biological, psychogeneological and energetic. German new medicine, biological decoding, bioneuroemotion and other similar schools are also based on identifying what they've called the "biological significance" of each organ, apparatus or system and its interaction with our biology. We've also already discussed transgenerational, family systemic and energetic references. Each of these can provide a perspective and a starting point for individual research.

It can be valuable to use the ideas of these various authors and researchers who've worked out their own catalogues of meanings, based on their experience and studies. Each contributes from their own point of reference, and they often complement each other. Personally, I'm inclined to start by listening to my own body. That's why I invite you, beyond offering a theoretical approach, to first feel things in your own body. It's a true privilege to be able to transcend what happens to us and reach another level of inquiry that leads directly to our center.

When you search for your own metaphor and then complement it with information from the aforementioned experts, it can be powerful. Of course, sometimes what you read from others may not seem to make sense. But remember, the full truth isn't necessarily on the conscious plane. Give yourself time to discover. Give space in your heart to those different points of view, noticing any resonance. Dialogue with one's own body is enriching and supports the search for that unique truth that may be the first step toward understanding how we got sick.

My chief interest is to stimulate self-inquiry. I want you to proceed in a spirit of becoming the primary investigator of yourself. Also, I hope that in the face of whatever happens to you, that you ask questions such as, "What do I want to say with this? What's the message for me? What do I have to learn? What screams at me from my body?" Even just asking these questions allows you to start down a different road. Invite the answers to begin to appear. This is already a big step toward taking responsibility for managing your own life.

To look for the message of an illness through questions like these doesn't mean that medical treatment may not be necessary or that general guidelines for health no longer apply. My point is that a person with a disease who maintains a good diet, applies medical prescriptions and specific therapies, seeks a quality lifestyle, is attuned to nature and on top of all that also investigates the message of a disease, this person has the opportunity not only to cure, but to heal. And in my experience, those who understand the importance of finding the cause behind an event (i.e. the message behind the illness), these are people for whom things flow in a different way.

CORRESPONDENCES FROM TRADITIONAL CHINESE MEDICINE (TCM)

TCM is where I first encountered the concept that emotions impact the physical structure and vice versa, as well as specific references to that which is expressed beyond the physical. It's thanks to TCM that I began to relate differently to my body and my patients. So I'll begin a list of correspondences from that tradition.

TCM looks at the being in its totality, maintaining the perspective that a person must be seen in the context of their environment, how they live, what happens to them, their emotions, thoughts and spirituality. It's also a tradition that views the human body as a wise receptacle of intelligent energies that sustain intracellular and organic life while maintaining a connection with everything around it. TCM speaks of a microcosm and a macrocosm and that, by a law of correspondences, we can link what is within the human being with all that exists at other levels of manifestation. These correspondences arise from profound observation of the changes and phenomena of nature, the seasons, the circadian cycle, the movements of the earth, the elements and their manifestations, and other knowledge. It's the idea that we can observe that which occurs outside to illuminate what also occurs within.

TCM led me to speak differently with patients and to pay intention to what was behind their reactions. By this, I mean that which is called *shen*, which is mental or psychic energy. *shen* is a Chinese term that can be translated in various ways, such as "spirit," "consciousness" or "psyche." It corresponds more to the Western concept of the mind. It's the most subtle way in which our energy or *qi* is expressed.

Shen has been considered the rector of consciousness. Accordingly, it's credited with the ability to recognize thoughts and feelings and the capacity of perception, including how we understand and react to stimuli. It is said in TCM that when the *shen* is calm and the perception is clear, the being raises its level of consciousness. This is why it is linked to the regulation of our capacity for self-knowledge and self-recognition. *Shen* is also related to the quality of sleep. If the *shen* is calm and balanced, the person will sleep well.

The heart *shen* is considered to be responsible for our projects and the dreams that become our life's purpose through the infusion of the emotional energy of the liver *(hum)*. The heart *shen* also energetically regulates the functions of the five senses: hearing, sight, touch, taste and smell. The heart *shen* also performs the very important function of coordinating and integrating the different parts of our mental and emotional life into an individual whole.

In Western medicine, most of the functions described above are attributed to the brain. That's why, in the context of TCM, the translation of *shen* as the "mind" may be much closer.

Each of the principal emotions in TCM is associated with an organ. Therefore, if you have a strong and sustained emotion, the organ or group of organs linked to that emotion can be affected. Here's a list of correlations between emotions, moods and different organs of the body, according to TCM:

ENERGY OF WATER	Fear. Responsibility. Insecurity. Trust. Courage.	These relate to the kidneys, bladder, bones, hair, the genital-urinary system, blood formation, hearing and the lumbar region.
ENERGY OF WOOD	Anger. Irritation. Intolerance. Tolerance. Tranquility. Decision.	These relate to the liver, gallbladder, tendons, muscles, ligaments and the sight.
ENERGY OF FIRE	Happiness. Sadness. Boredom. Apathy. Creativity.	These relate to the heart, small intestine, circulatory system and speech.
ENERGY OF EARTH	Reflection. Worry. Obsession. Doubt. Skepticism. Good mood.	These relate to the spleen, stomach, pancreas, the sense of taste and distribution of flavors.
ENERGY OF METAL	Sadness. Depression. Attachment. Fullness. Satisfaction. Nostalgia. Melancholy.	These relate to the lungs, large intestine, skin, hair, throat and upper respiratory system.

Here's an example. If a person accumulates a lot of anger for a long time, eventually it will begin to affect their liver, initially causing an energetic imbalance. Naturally, the question of whether or not the person later develops or manifests a physical illness or imbalance depends on multiple other variables that can coexist. Still, this ancient concept connecting emotions and organs once again illustrates the importance of treating the person as a whole.

I've had impressive experiences along these lines, both personally and with patients. For instance, with detoxifications of the liver, I've seen several cases where a person has begun to release their anger and, with a little extra help, they've been able to free themselves from old grudges and feelings of helplessness that had long been serious issues for them. Some of these patients had previously tried purely psychological and emotional methods of treatment and been unable to shift the emotion. The therapy helped somewhat but the anger continued to return. And I'm talking about people who'd done both personal and spiritual work but were still struggling to manage their anger. Their irritability was in full bloom. By accepting my suggestion of a detox – which is what the body was asking for – they were able to achieve the needed emotional release. Fundamentally, this is a dual approach. By working with the emotions, the body begins to get better. By working on the body with specific treatments of particular areas, we can help unlock related emotions.

OTHER CORRESPONDENCES OF CORPORAL TOPOGRAPHY

In any given reading of the body we can find several possible correspondences. These will depend on the references (repressed emotions, energetic blockages, early traumas, ancestral inheritances, etc.) and different sources may suggest different correspondences. Also, the information must be adapted to the individual and their experiences. Once again, the physical symptoms are calls to attention.

From this perspective, our build, gestures and bodily characteristics become sublime and subtle messages that can be applied to the internal maps we make for how we move through life. These messages can be further revealed through postures, ways of walking, whatever parts of the body we push forward, our axes of balance and support and so on.

I've collected a number of possible correlations, according to my own experience and associations I've been able to make, as well as from various references encountered through my training, professional relationships and from books by various authors. I'm also drawing on information from German new medicine, biological decoding and other approaches that give "biological meanings" to emotional distress. There are no recipes for this and it's not meant as a rigid pattern.

LATERALITY

Laterality (the dominance of one side over the other) is significant, quite aside from the organ in question. What do our halves say?

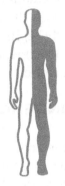

MASCULINE ENERGY

(Right side of the body)

Corresponds to *yang* energy, the masculine, the relationship with the father and men. Also with the external, the outside, expression, the expansive, action, giving and the intellectual plane.

FEMININE ENERGY

(Left side of the body)

Corresponds to *yin* energy, the feminine, the relationship with the mother and women. Also with the eternal, the inside, introspection, stillness, receiving, welcoming, emotions, creativity and the intuitive.

ANCESTRY

In working with the family tree, as previously mentioned, the idea is that the strata of our family tree exists in each of our bodies. This can be expressed roughly as follows:

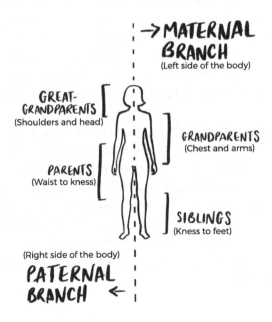

→ **MATERNAL BRANCH**
(Left side of the body)

GREAT-GRANDPARENTS
(Shoulders and head)

GRANDPARENTS
(Chest and arms)

PARENTS
(Waist to kness)

SIBLINGS
(Kness to feet)

(Right side of the body)
PATERNAL BRANCH ←

MORE REFERENCES

At the back of this book I've included an appendix with further observations that may shed light on the corporal topography of certain conditions. It's a brief reference guide which each person can adjust or adapt to their own reality and perception.

A FINAL MESSAGE ABOUT ALL DISEASES

Ultimately, it doesn't really matter how a sickness was initiated or whether or not the physical or emotional cause is even discovered. Your discomfort gives you the suggestion to return to your heart and the message is: Love yourself!

Love allows you to direct your process from the heart and not from reason alone. Through self-love, you give yourself permission to reconnect and do whatever you decide without judging yourself or further self-punishment. Then you can fully bring yourself to accept that your human parts are full of fears, pains, limiting beliefs, grudges, envy, laziness, pride, vanity and attachments. You can accept your weaknesses as well as your strengths and comfort zones without abusing yourself any more. From a place of recognition and respect, you can make the leap to another level of consciousness where your shadows and your lights commune.

With self-love you can appreciate the road you've traveled even if you don't feel proud of everything you've done to get where you are. Loving recognition allows you to thank and forgive others and yourself, and this gives a boost to your healing. You can also then look on others and their journeys with respect. It is indeed possible to live without judgement. In fact, it opens the way for a healthier coexistence, first with yourself and then with others.

Self-love also allows you to see your responsibility and make the changes you need in a fluid way, instead of seeing those changes as punishment or impositions. Instead, they become a beautiful opportunity to both give and receive what you've denied yourself. And you can do so with gratitude, realizing you have the opportunity to act, to breathe with a greater connection and consciousness of life, even to reach something more spiritual. As the Chinese proverb says, "Nothing feels better to the body than growth of the spirit."

Self-love allows you to connect with everyone and everything else, including your illness. Love is a powerful medicine and it begins with you!

PART III

REMOVE

**THE ART OF LIVING IMPLIES
KNOWING WHEN TO HOLD ON
AND WHEN TO LET GO.**

HEVELOCK ELLIS

CHAPTER 14

REMOVE: BET ON A DETOXIFIED LIFE

"To fly higher, life doesn't take things from you, it frees you from them . . ."

— ANONYMOUS

Maybe your life is stagnant, paralyzed, or you have a lot of potential and you can't seem to set it in motion. Or maybe you have feelings that undermine your well-being and development. These might be grudges, self-criticism, fears, anger, deep unprocessed pain or limiting fears of scarcity. Maybe you're suffering from a chronic, degenerative disease. Or you have symptoms, pains and ailments that don't match your age. Or maybe your vitality is just not what it was. Frankly, with any of these reasons it may benefit you to make a plan of detoxification.

Likewise, if everything's fine and you simply want to reinforce your health, I propose a "life detox." Remember that my general approach includes prevention as the best of options to bring your life to an optimal state and make the most of your potential. This is why you can experience detox as a regular scheduled process or as a way of life in which you stay as non-toxic as possible.

Remove generates a discharge. It's as if we were walking through life with a heavy pack on our backs that we've carried so long, we're accustomed to it. Now we consciously undo the straps and take it off and as we do, we realize we can walk better without it. We can focus our energy better and be more productive.

There's always something to let go, even if you're not going through a crisis or at a point where you're feeling stuck. It's healthy to periodically check your physical spaces, the body, the emotional closet and the toxic thoughts of the moment and find a way to lighten and free them. Detoxify yourself periodically at every level: physical, mental and emotional.

In a therapeutic process this phase usually comes after the *Review* (unless there are specific conditions that prevent it). Once the life or medical history has been recorded and the therapist has a clear idea of the patient's background, interference, emotional readings, blockages and toxins at different levels, the next step is to plan the *Remove*. This is part of "preparing the ground," a metaphor borrowed from agriculture. It's how a farmer readies the soil before planting. The ground is weeded, tilled and plowed so the seeds are sown in better soil. Preparing the ground before sowing makes all the difference at harvest time. Likewise, it makes the body more receptive and responsive.

To the extent that we detoxify ourselves physically, emotionally or mentally, we can nourish, repair, rebuild and revitalize more favorably. *Remove* can help clear the connection between mind, body and emotions in general. It can also help you lose weight if you need to and lighten your body. Most importantly, it helps renew and maintain strong internal resistance, so you can respond much better to any other treatment, therapy or necessary procedure.

CHAPTER 15

PHYSICAL DETOXIFICATION

*"From now on, I just want to carry what's in my pocket
and in my heart."*

— ANONYMOUS

To purify the body is to decrease its level of toxemia. One way this is done is by decreasing our contact with elements that are toxic to the system. The other way it's done is by helping the eliminating organs to perform their function, stimulating the drainage of toxins.

The health of an individual depends to a great extent on the ability of his or her body to dispose of harmful residues, both from internal and external origins. The body has organs and systems responsible for cleaning up impurities and organic wastes. These are the liver, kidneys, skin, the intestines and the lungs. Elimination occurs through sweat, air, feces, urine, lymph and the lymphatic system. This is normal physiology. The waste of the food is expelled from the cells and passes into the lymph and blood, which transport it to the excretory organs, especially the liver and the kidneys, where it's transformed and moved to the organs of evacuation.

The human organism is actually designed to purify itself and is constantly purging naturally. It detoxifies substances from the metabolic waste produced by the body itself and also from toxic substances from outside. The speed and effectiveness with which these processes occur depend the age of the person, their level of interior preservation or deterioration (particularly the organs most involved in purification) and also the accumulation of pollutants through exposure. In other words, although the body has a natural waste recycling system, it can fail to some degree in cases where the body has over-exceeded the limits it can tolerate. Unfortunately, in our modern era this tends to happen quite often. We're in contact with a variety of organic and inorganic substances that end up circulating inside us and many are deposited in the inner layers of the tissues. These hinder the normal functioning of our organs.

There are many elements that are classified as toxic or that act as such when entering the body in large quantities. The most common are found in: preservatives and chemicals in foods, gardening products, cosmetics, body lotions, deodorants, toothpastes, hair products, kitchen utensils, detergents and cleaning products, byproducts of fumigation, the byproducts of industrial activity, hydrocarbons from internal combustion engines, batteries, additives to purify water, plastic containers, and on and on. Few people realize the quantity of environmental and household pollutants we're exposed to that are considered "normal." We can control or minimize our exposure to some of these toxic substances but there are some we can't, especially if we live in urban areas.

We've come to understand the harm caused by free radicals. These are toxic metabolic waste substances that damage the body and are not directly eliminated. A healthy person can handle the presence of free radicals by defending the body with their own anti-free radical system. However, if the amount of free radicals produced by the body is greater than our physiological and biological processes can counteract, the end result is oxidative stress that causes cellular damage.

Aside from many of the environment pollutants already mentioned, the production of free radicals is mainly stimulated by stress, alcohol, tobacco, processed foods, drugs, saturated fats, fried foods, sugars (especially refined sugar), artificial preservatives and other additives that improve the taste, color or consistency of food. There are also pollutants generated through the processing, packaging and storage of various goods.

It's also worthwhile listing here the five foods that many specialists in integrative health have labelled The Five Metabolic Poisons. They are sugar, refined flour, salt, white rice and milk. These five foods are the primary physical inducers of many degenerative and inflammatory diseases such as arthritis, diabetes, cancer, heart problems, colitis, vascular insufficiencies, premature aging and more.

With our lack of control over polluting agents, our polluted food and our sedentary, stressed lives, our level of toxic overload is generally very high. So it becomes increasingly difficult for the body to deal with it all and stay balanced at the same time. This ends up creating the right biological environment for various degenerative diseases, many of which are fatal.

The detoxifying process of the body begins by cleansing and restoring the function of the gastrointestinal tract, primarily using changes in the diet and purification practices. Then the detoxifying systems of the liver and kidneys activate. Finally, the toxins deposited in the tissues and cells are purified. In short, all of our vital organs and processes of elimination are stimulated. This is necessary when treating any condition, but especially degenerative ones.

In addition to dietary changes, the body's natural process can be aided with certain practices and therapies. These are not new techniques. They come from ancient medical traditions and have long been used for both acute and chronic diseases. Some of these are regular practices for a less toxic lifestyle. Others are methods and treatment plans for specific situations. When we detoxify the body, we promote creativity, motivation and productivity. Our available energy increases, and we enhance our relaxation. This allows for better rest and greater health for our vital organs and skin and it slows cellular aging.

One of the most important aspects of maximizing the effect of your physical detox is mental preparation. It requires a firm commitment to carry out a detox program. Your focus and discipline are crucial to greater success. Going through the process with greater awareness will also help you connect more with the sense of being integrated. It can help you enter into a state of greater coherence and presence. That's been my experience. I'm happy to relate that in my personal program of detox with a dual physical and emotional purpose, the results have been very powerful.

You prepare yourself better for the challenges that arise in the process when you're aware of the benefits and you know why you do it. You visualize yourself healthier and more vital, so you include that sense of purpose in the process. The challenges include your appetites and the temptation for things you're giving up, especially addictive foods like sweets. Other challenges may include symptoms that appear as a result of removing toxins and making dietary changes. These symptoms can be physical or emotional: headaches, constipation, diarrhea, flatulence, skin eruptions, a cough, a stronger body odor, anxiety, irritability, depression, insomnia and more. With any type of addiction this step may represent an even tougher challenge. In such cases, it may be more appropriate to undertake with greater supervision.

You may also need to prepare for the discouraging or skeptical opinions of those who try to get you to abandon the whole thing. These drain your energy.

Keeping a diary can be a useful part of the process and can enrich it. You can record your physical symptoms, emotional symptoms, new awareness, small victories and dreams,

One way to begin is to eliminate any foods from your regular diet with artificial coloring or sugars, as well as soft drinks, canned goods, fried foods, artificial flavorings (including canned sauces, diced flavorings or seasonings), reused oils, added sugar and artificial sweeteners, fast food, processed and junk food. Also, you can reduce your consumption of salt, juices, cheeses, saturated fats (custard, margarine, sweet cream, pâté), sausages, refined flour (white bread, cookies, pasta, wheat tortillas), ice cream, pastry, sweets and excess caffeine, alcohol and tobacco. With all this, you will already have begun to stimulate the internal biological processes and to promote a more vital diet.

There are many examples of toxic elements in what we consume daily. Some, such as mercury, arsenic, lead, pesticides, dioxins and hormones, end up in our foods through the process of production. Others are added through the food industry's processing: dyes, preservatives (BHA and BHT, potassium bromate, sodium nitrates), flavorings, and bisphenol (BPA) from some food containers. There are others.

However, simply changing your diet is not enough to detoxify, especially if you've abused your system with toxic habits for a long time. It's also often necessary to do something more. For example, you could do a stronger, more specific cleansing to mark the beginning of a new daily health routine. TCM suggests a periodic, seasonal cleansing for prevention in the spring and fall. These seasons are particularly conducive to the activity of organs such as the liver, gallbladder, large intestine, lungs and the skin, all of which are said to be physiologically involved in elimination. You can also keep a regular exercise routine, take steam baths, do breathing and relaxation exercises, get massages for relaxation and lymphatic drainage and get enough rest. You can also go to the sea or the mountains and breathe cleaner air. Bear in mind though, that with certain purification processes, such as special programs for impaired health conditions, I suggest doing so under medical supervision.

Coffee Enemas

I learned the benefits of coffee enemas when I studied orthomolecular nutrition. Eventually I made them part of my personal health routine and began prescribing them to patients.

Enemas are a very old practice, but the notion reemerged among the cancer therapy measures suggested by Dr. Max Gerson in the 1930s. Gerson proposed the practice of coffee enemas based on his conviction that the caffeine stimulates the liver and gallbladder to release and detoxify. His work has been continued by his daughter, Charlotte Gerson, who in 1978 founded the Gerson Institute, an internationally known center for the natural treatment of cancer.

In 1981, Dr. Lee Wattenberg and his colleagues were in fact able to demonstrate that substances found in coffee, including palmitic acids, stimulate the production of the enzyme glutathione s-transferase, promoting liver purification.[26]

Regular organic coffee enemas were one of my partners in overcoming cancer. They continue to be an important health practice for me, and they've become a space of peace and quiet; indeed, of intimacy. First, I take the time to prepare the physical space: a clean bathroom, relaxing music and half-light. I create an atmosphere that helps me to spend the time in introspection or silence. I turn it into a *welcoming womb*. During the process, I take the opportunity to visualize, to pray, to send messages of gratitude to my body or love to my cells. I channel my creativity into my health. I put myself in the mental and emotional frame of mind to break free from old patterns or from lingering conscious or unconscious feelings that hinder me from fulfilling my purpose.

I share my personal experience with coffee enemas in the hope that it motivates you to do your purging from this kind of perspective. I assure you, you can move beyond the mental discomfort that arises at the mere suggestion. The discomfort or awkwardness of applying a coffee enema is part of the beginning of the process, but once you adapt it becomes comfortable as well as beneficial.

CHAPTER 16

FASTING AS A WAY OF PURIFYING

"Food, in convalescence, strengthens; in sickness, it weakens."

— HIPPOCRATES

It's become somewhat unpopular, but fasting is a personal practice that's been very beneficial for me. It's also been a catalyst for many insights and helped me develop discipline. Along with its detoxifying effect, fasting can facilitate health maintenance and help improve multiple conditions. Fasting aids in the restoration of cells and has been observed to have an effect on the elongation of telomeres (compound structures which protect the ends of chromosomes. I'll discuss telomeres in Chapters 21 and 22).

To fast is to abstain from ingesting food for a period of time, but it's much more than just not eating. Fasting is a conscious, voluntary act of renouncing not just food, but all kinds of compulsive or automatic behaviors. It's not a new practice either. For thousands of years, in both Eastern and Western cultures, periods of fasting were a regular practice. Fasting was used with the triple intention of bodily cleansing, mental decontamination and spiritual clarity. It was also practiced before performing tasks involving strength, concentration or emotional stability.

There are biblical accounts of fasting and it was also among the therapeutic practices of the Egyptians. It was routinely practiced in ancient Greece. Plato and Socrates fasted regularly to stimulate mental and physical clarity. In the Hippocratic model, food restraint was a rule for acute illness. Hippocrates and Paracelsus considered fasting as an essential practice to enhance our self-healing capacity, so much so that Paracelsus referred to it as the most powerful remedy.

When we fast, according to Dahlke and Dethlefsen, the "inner physician" interacts with the organism and we give ourselves an experience that completely purifies soul and body and even, in certain cases, brings us to a new level of life.[27]

Fasting gives the organism a physiological rest. It promotes healing by setting in motion all the mechanisms of detoxification, regeneration and self-regulation. The energy that was being used in digestion and the assimilation of nutrients is channeled to the processes of elimination. Nothing is lost that's vital. What's lost is not useful: excessive fat, including cholesterol, long-accumulated toxic waste substances and the like.

Fasting stimulates liver restoration and muscle tonicity of the stomach and intestines. It recuperates the peristaltic movements, revitalizes the pancreas and heart and stimulates the immune system. The anti-inflammatory effect promotes greater health and in general benefits all the tissues of the body.

The completion of a long fast provides a special opportunity to reorganize eating habits and move toward a better quality diet. It serves as a starting point for a renewed program that optimizes health.

From another perspective, eating and fasting go together like sleep and keeping a vigil, breathing in and breathing out. They are a duality, two poles that are part of the same natural rhythm.

Most people can receive the benefits of fasting. However, it's contraindicated in cases of pregnancy and lactation, renal failure, severe heart disease, diabetes, hypoglycemia, cirrhosis of the liver, extreme thinness or cachexia, very advanced cancerous tumors, stomach or duodenal ulcer, for patients with organ transplants.

INTERMITTENT FASTING

This kind of fasting involves alternating periods of fasting and feeding. Among the various possible schedules, the best-known are fasting 16/8, fasting 24, fasting 48, or fasting 12/12. A 16/8 fast consists of abstaining from food for 16 hours followed by a feeding period of 8 hours. So if we eat a first meal at 1:00 p.m., the intake of all our food is in the 8 hours between 1:00 and 9:00 p.m., with two meals during that time. The next day we eat again at 1 p.m., 16 hours from the previous meal. Fasting 24 and 48 are based on periods of abstention of 24 and 48 hours, respectively.

Intermittent fasting is a good strategy for a person who should ingest less calories. It allows the calories to be grouped into just one or two meals.

For a person used to having many meals a day, my suggestion is to first reduce your number of meals to three (breakfast, lunch and dinner). Once you've adopted this routine, the next step is to reduce your breakfast calories to such an extent that breakfast doesn't count. Then it will be relatively simple to cut down to just two meals a day. The next step of trying a 24-hour fast should then be easy.

For those who want to gain muscle mass, it all depends on one's type of metabolism. If it's slow and you can gain weight by minimally increasing caloric consumption, intermittent fasting is also a good strategy.

Intermittent fasting has multiple benefits. It can adjust our metabolic health, regulating insulin resistance, which also positively affects the telomeres. It delays aging by reducing oxidative stress. It reduces the indicators of inflammation and may even limit the growth of cancer cells. It balances the lipid profile and has positive effects on brain plasticity.

Mark Mattson is a veteran researcher at the National Institute of Aging, a branch of the U.S. National Institutes of Health (NIH). Mattson has investigated the health benefits of intermittent fasting and says that "during a period of fasting, the cells are under mild stress and respond to adaptive tension by improving their ability to deal with stress and, perhaps, to resist disease. There is a considerable similarity between how cells respond to exercise stress and how cells respond to intermittent fasting."[28]

Adequate nutrition becomes even more impactful when fasting. It's advisable to identify your dietary choices before starting a fast. This includes minimizing carbohydrates and replacing them with healthy fats, such as coconut oil, olive oil, olives, *ghee* (a clarified butter), avocados and nuts. Also, consider the suggestions I've made to ingest a minimal level of toxins.

Individual conditions, however, must be taken into account for any kind of fast and it's best to consult your family doctor to make sure it's safe for you and to determine what kind of fast best suits your physical situation and state of health.

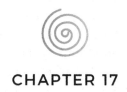

CHAPTER 17

TOXINS IN YOUR ENVIRONMENT

"Sometimes less is more."

— ANONYMOUS

Remove extends to the physical spaces where you live and work. This means getting rid of things you no longer use or serve a purpose. It means freeing up spaces that may be useful for something else or simply giving yourself more room to breathe. It's a physical cleansing but it also has greater repercussions.

There's a universal principle from Hermetic philosophy that says, "As above so below; as within so without." That which we feel and think, we reflect on the outside. The richness or poverty of our mind and heart translates into the flow of our external lives.

Changing our mentality, our attitudes, our impulses and conditioning doesn't happen overnight. It requires recognition and then a sustained plan of observation and action to modify our sense of flow and abundance. Just as we can't instantly detoxify the body, this process takes time.

Cleaning your physical spaces is a good way to accompany another type of detox or any new beginning. You can begin with something as simple as cleaning out and giving away things you've stored for so long you hardly remember you have them. In the same way that you keep clothes and other objects "just in case" or have overloaded closets or shelves of books, you spend your life accumulating unmade decisions, unspoken words, affections unexpressed, unresolved formalities, emotional receipts, expired thoughts and toxins in the body. Too often these things go hand in hand and the congestion hinders the free flow of your life.

All that you accumulate is what stagnates you, what holds you back and becomes an impediment. It's not just the objects themselves, it's the attitude behind the habit of accumulating. That state of mind that makes us keep a piece of clothing or equipment we don't need or use is the same one that won't allow our emotions to flow or won't allow us to resolve a problem of resentment or economic deprivation.

The external practice of *Remove*, in addition to making our space more alive, generates places for new things to come and helps us connect with the force and consciousness of that which flows. There's abundance for all in the universe. It's up to us to receive and accept it.

Moving, circulating, eliminating or recycling can change our attitude of attachment or clinging to things, which is nothing more than the fear of not having, the fear of scarcity. But just that fear connects us with more scarcity, because then that's how we vibrate. It's what we attract. The message we send our unconscious is of lack, mistrust, attachment to the past or being undeserving. It's as if the new and better doesn't correspond to us. We send our cells a message of poverty, of poor functioning. It's a message of low vitality, stagnation and the impossibility of change.

By unburdening, materially and emotionally, we attract more easily what we desire. We enter into the energy of prosperity and healing. We flow with a life that's characterized by movement and we fill ourselves with vitality. Our cells are revitalized, we recover the brightness in our eyes which expresses an inner strength.

So, go to it! Get into gear: clean, dust, clear away cobwebs inside and out so you continue to flow with life and in connection with your sense of abundance and renewal. Also, as we talk about cleaning our spaces, I want to discuss another fundamental aspect. From ancient times to the present, the relationship of human society to the environment has varied greatly, but the level of pollution we currently generate is appalling, with far more serious consequences to our health than we often realize. Much of this is industrial pollution generated through the production of products for consumption. As part of the macro-environment in which we all breathe and work, these poisons are potentially as influential as our family micro-environment. They reach the intimacy of the cellular environment. This is of course a broad topic with many facets, but taking it to the practical level for day to day feasibility, I want to share a few suggestions to make your immediate environment more clean and safe.

Most of the conventional cleaning products we grew up with contain petroleum products with colorants and other additives with dubious implications for our health and the environment. There are more and more brands of healthy, ecological and effective products to keep a house clean and smelling fresh. Many of these products are non-toxic, biodegradable and made of renewable resources, as opposed to petroleum products. There are also various household staples that can be used for cleaning. Vinegar and baking soda can clean almost anything.

Antibacterial and antimicrobial soaps don't necessarily clean hands better than regular soap and water, plus they increase the risk of breeding "super germs" (bacteria impervious to disinfectants). The USFDA (U.S. Food and Drug Administration) has affirmed that antibacterial soaps and hand cleaners do not work better than normal soap and water and recommends that they be avoided for routine, household use.

Be careful with synthetic air fresheners. Instead, try boiling cinnamon, cloves or another herb you like. Use therapeutic grade essential oils. They will not only give you a pleasant aroma, they can also help you as an antiseptic. I can recommend lemon, tea tree oil, cinnamon, lavender and cypress.

Also, plants may not make your house smell differently, but they're good for filtering the indoor air. Almost any plant with wide green leaves will do. Don't forget to open windows and even the doors of cabinets and drawers to ventilate them and allow the recycling of the air to help you maintain cleanliness.

Finally, when you replace cleaning products, don't just throw the old ones away. If they're too toxic for your home, they're too toxic to pour down the sink or toilet or simply put in the trash to go to the dump. There are safer options for their disposal.

The process of creating a green space is delicate and requires some re-education.

CHAPTER 18

THE MENTAL AND EMOTIONAL PURGE

"Releasing is oxygenating the soul."
— MOSHE DAYAN

Emotions a part of human nature; they allow you to relate to the world. But you have emotions that have been locked inside you since childhood. You've hidden feelings of fear, anger or sadness because maybe you were taught these were bad emotions and you fear disapproval. Even now you don't always process them well and they become toxins that keep you from keep you from moving forward easily and expressing the best of you. You can identify them through inappropriate or disproportionate reactions in your adult life.

Another major source of emotional toxins is stress. It's a source of physical toxins too, because under stress the body releases substances such as adrenaline, cortisol and others that raise the heart rate, increase blood pressure and alter the metabolism. If the stress is chronic and consistent, there can be an accumulation of hormones and metabolic residue that keep the inner environment toxic. This weakens the immune system in general, but it can also cause fatigue, headaches, allergies, skin disorders, depression, anxiety and other emotional imbalances.

Cleaning up your emotional home opens up the space for new experiences and a fuller state of being. The stagnant thoughts and emotions that couldn't be processed - resentment, anger, envy, fear, pain, betrayal, helplessness, and the like - are just as toxic and harmful as physical toxins, if not removed. There's no way to isolate them because we function as an interconnected whole with close ties.

Once you've identified emotions that you get caught up in and you realize how expert you've become at swallowing what you feel, it's time to release those feelings and move forward.

Learn to express your feelings without hurting. If you feel a lot of anger and it's not the right time or place to express it, give yourself time to calm down or choose an indirect method such as hitting a cushion, screaming under a pillow or squeezing a towel. Feel the rage all through your body, but let it out. If you notice fear overtaking you: give yourself permission to tremble. Feel it throughout your body until it passes. Don't avoid or ignore it. If you're very sad: cry, scream from your depths or seek out a person who can silently hug you with no judgment, simply offering to hold you as long as you need it.

It's important to release emotions both verbally and physically so the energy leaves the emotional and physical body. Releasing emotions verbally means talking about what happens to you and what makes you feel bad. It means honestly sharing your feelings with someone or even alone in front of a mirror, or talking to an empty chair or writing. Releasing emotions on the physical level means expressing yourself physically, like clenching your fists or shaking or contracting parts of the body.

Don't let yourself be poisoned by not knowing how to express your feelings. This is an art that's learned and perfected by practice. When we hold back or swallow our emotions they become ruminations in our thoughts and last longer than necessary.

If you become aware that you've been unable to fully let go of a feeling and find yourself in an ongoing painful emotional state, seek professional help. Allow yourself the support of healing in the company of a good professional. It's time to enjoy inner freedom and choose how you want to live.

FORGIVENESS AS AN ACT OF EMOTIONAL PURIFICATION

The path of forgiveness is not always easy and forgiving oneself is usually hardest of all. The guilt, the weight you carry in your heart with constant thoughts and memories of mistakes you've made is like a heavy load of rocks in your backpack. It's as if you were driving your car with the emergency brake engaged. It slows you down and hinders you.

You can get obsessed by ghosts of the past, shadows of past errors and things you regret. This turns guilt into your guide. You punish yourself, you fear the future and you don't in live the present. Guilt limits your vision of yourself as well as others. Of course, it's easy to simply say, "We all make mistakes in life." Guilt is a complex issue. But to be clear, I'm referring here only to conscious guilt for something we remember, not to systemic burdens where we unconsciously try to repair a family member's imbalance from the past or where we unconsciously shoulder burdens that our not ours. However, these situations are also common, where people act from an unconscious guilt that leads to a lack of self-worth.

The ways in which you haven't been able to forgive influence the choices you make and the possibilities you believe in. If you can't forgive, part of your inner life energy is trapped in resentment, anger, pain or suffering of some kind. This trapped vital energy limits you at every turn.

Learning to live with mistakes and knowing they're part of life itself will lead to forgiveness. As you forgive yourself, the energy that drifted into negative thoughts and feelings is set free. This lets down the resistance and limitations you've created, allowing you to move forward and to connect with your worthiness.

Through forgiveness, when you release your mental and emotional energies, you'll be able to maintain better relationships and manifest your true potential. The act of forgiveness requires a decision. Free yourself and let go with love and you will see great changes in your life. Forgiveness starts with you. Forgive yourself first!

CHAPTER 19

THE GRIEF IN SICKNESS

"Nothing confronts us more with the true meaning of life than the possibility of losing it."

– ANONYMOUS

Grief is the consequence of a loss. It's a process of adapting to something that's no longer there, the emptiness of a broken link. There are varied reactions to dealing with the stress that follows a significant loss. These include emotional, social and physical changes at different levels.

When someone speaks of grieving, most people – including you, probably – immediately think of the loss of a loved one. But we can also grieve the loss of work, grown children leaving the house, the death of a pet, retirement, and so on.

The issue of grief has been written about a great deal at the psychotherapeutic level. More people every day turn to a therapist or counselor to help them process a loss. This is an accompaniment of active listening that helps lay the emotions on the table to talk about them, validate them and gradually put them in a good place. When you look them in the face, these things are less menacing.

What I want to focus on here is another kind of grief, a kind which isn't often taken into account. That's the grief related to the loss of physical health.

Before continuing, I think it's worth repeating that sometimes grief can be hidden, repressed in the unconscious until something triggers it. Then when it comes to the surface it can generate another subsequent grief.

Diseases often produce a physical surprise. A disease appears and suddenly you miss what was lost: your health. This shock is stronger with catastrophic illnesses and accidents in which a person is disfigured. This might be the loss of a body part, an amputation, the loss of one of the senses, mobility or another function, or any significant change in the person's appearance and general condition. The aftermath of an accident leaves marks on the emotions as well as the body. We're a unified body-mind, so when a person is confronted with the misfortune of losing their health, the physical pain is joined by psychic pain.

The person in these cases passes through stages similar to the stages of mourning the loss a loved one. There's the loss in itself. Then there's the denial ("It's not possible. This can't be happening to me, not now . . ."). Then comes anger, sometimes accompanied by indictment ("It's not fair, It's not right, I neglected, I didn't realize . . ."). Next comes fear for what's coming, or might happen and how to face it. The layers of pain and sadness can be deep.

In the midst of these raw emotions it's important to validate them, to give oneself space to experience them physically and to express them. Giving yourself permission to feel, even to collapse, is part of self-respect and validation. To vent the pain, to cry or scream it or speak it from your deepest feelings is human and restorative. As I've said, letting the pain pass through your body and express itself is surrendering to what Eckhart Tolle and others have called the "body of pain."

Later comes the ascent, when you gradually emerge from the shock and begin a shift toward reparation and hope. This comes with acceptance, with making peace with the loss and looking forward to something positive in the time to come. This is what allows us to move on to the phase *Resignify*, where we are able to see the lesson, the hidden message in our loss. To receive the gift of the pain. To *Resignify* is to recognize what we've done in response to our loss and it demonstrates our courage. We come to a place where we can evoke what happened in peace.

To live with grief consciously is also a way of yielding to something willingly rather than holding on to the feeling that life is "cheating" you. It lifts you out of the role of the victim and allows you to take into your hands that which is yours.

This process is not linear. There are many theories that describe it in a more or less similar way. I choose this way of describing it based on my own griefs and the processes I've experienced with patients, some of whom had lost loved ones and many of whom were dealing with the loss of an organ.

The purpose of the experience of grief is to be able to appreciate life regardless of what's been lost, however threatening it may be. No matter the circumstance, saying *yes* to life is necessary to continue and to find resilience.

CHAPTER 20

DIGITAL DETOX

*"The most important contact is the one you have
with yourself when you tune in to the heart."*

— RAQUELINA LUNA

A few years back, when I started thinking about writing this
book, digital detox was not a topic that occurred to me. But
we live now in such a technological, digital world, I think
not including the subject would leave out an increasingly
relevant health concern.

We're in the age of instant communication. Most of
us have a smartphone, a PC or laptop, a tablet or all of the
above. I wonder every day what technology can do. I'm
an active user of technology, though I don't consider myself savvy and I generally underuse my very sophisticated
equipment. Still, I try to keep up with the best ways to benefit from these resources and I happily use them for my work
and my personal life.

Clearly, I support the use of technology. At the same
time, I've occasionally found myself in a state of what I call
hyper-communication. It's like, wherever I go, people can
access me or I can access them and it's almost inconceivable
that I wouldn't instantly answer a message. It's hard to disconnect. I've come to feel completely dependent on walking

with my phone and if I don't have it, it's as if something important is missing and I don't like that feeling.

There are groups of people at tables everywhere, each with a cell phone. If they stop looking at their phone for a moment, it's only to take a picture to post on social media, and that's no exaggeration. Families, couples, friends and colleagues eat in a restaurant, each with their phone next to their plate and they're more attentive to their phones than to sharing with each other. The common denominator is their mobile equipment, with everything in miniature: the telephone itself, the agenda, the camera, access to email, social networks, electronic games, search engines and chats. Oh, the chats!

One issue is the dependence on constant communication and the compulsion to constantly review what's happening in the world or to send information to others. The other issue is the over-exposure to the electro-magnetic emissions of the machines themselves. The worst part of that is that many people sleep with their phones practically glued to them, under their pillow or on the nightstand, close to their heads. There's still a lot of disinformation about electro-magnetic emissions and we don't fully know the real consequences. They're masked by other pollutants. But electro-magnetic pollution is a reality and we're overexposed to it.

I won't go into the subject of antennas or Wi-Fi. I'm leaving that as homework for myself. But for the time being, let's take both factors into account: direct exposure through our ears and bodies, and the behavioral addiction to being constantly connected.

Finally, the so-called age of communication is a relative term. Close communication hasn't necessarily improved and dialogue hasn't necessarily opened. The *magic* of our machines absorbs and traps us and we miss the possibility of relating to those in front of us. Worse still, we lose the connection with ourselves. We lose the ability to be alone, to be in real silence, to really concentrate on things and to be more present in our lives.

This is a broad topic but it's worth considering what we should be asking, and even more, what we should be doing. The first thing is to become aware of your reality with digital communication, the justifications you have to be constantly engaged, bordering on an obsessive need. What if you suddenly decide not to keep checking? Does it make you impatient? Can you stand it? Do you make up an excuse to just go ahead and check? Do you think you're missing something really important?

I invite you to consider the following suggestions, which I've named the Digital Detox Diet.

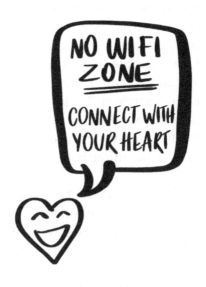

ACTIONS FOR A R.E.A.L. LIFE

DIGITAL DETOX DIET

Don't walk around on weekends with your cell phone all the time.

Every once in a while, schedule a retreat time: no phone, no emails, no chats, etc. If necessary, announce to others (by the same means) that you won't be available for a few hours (or more) and that you'll be offline.

Avoid leaving your cell phone next to your bed before you sleep. If you use it as an alarm (that was my excuse for a time), buy a little battery alarm clock and put it on your nightstand.

Eat quietly: not in front of the TV or computer, and no phone.

Disable notifications and alerts from social networks and emails, as they disrupt your concentration, distract you and increase your need to keep checking. This is especially important at work, when you drive and when you're in groups.

Turn off your Wi-Fi at night before bed and turn it back on when you need it, so you avoid unnecessary radiation and contribute to a cleaner environment.

Share these concerns with your friends. Ask them to join your detox program. Talk about what happens to you and share it in groups.

PART IV

REPAIR

**THE NATURAL FORCES
THAT ARE WITHIN US
ARE THE TRUE HEALERS OF
DISEASE.**

HIPPOCRATES

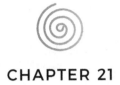

CHAPTER 21

REPAIR: AWAKEN YOUR GIFT OF REGENERATION

"What you do today can improve every morning."
— RALPH MARSTON

After removing and releasing toxic elements from the body and the being, it's time to *Repair* the overall system. The verb *repair* refers to "fixing something that's broken or damaged," "amending, correcting or remedying," and "reestablishing strength, giving breath or vigor." This is precisely what happens at this stage. It fixes, corrects and resets forces that aren't working optimally. It reconnects the vital flow.

The *Repair* phase is intended to restore the body to the best possible health conditions. In mild cases, such as individuals with good physical responses and their systems intact, once initial steps are taken (detoxification, changes in diet, exercise and some energetic therapy), the body begins to react positively right away. Sometimes it doesn't take much more than discipline and perseverance to eventually achieve remarkable and sustainable change.

As part of the normal physiological process of the body our cells are constantly multiplying. Every tissue has its own rhythm of renewal but all of our cells are replaced in an orderly process of multiplication every seven years or so. Then we have a "new" body.

At the cellular level, regeneration involves restoring or replacing our body's damaged or aged cells and tissues, because otherwise they won't function optimally. Even though as we age our cells regenerate more slowly, we can still facilitate this process to a significant extent.

When a cell suffers damage, naturally and spontaneously the mechanisms of repair immediately begin to act to avoid irreversible damage. But this ability can slow and stagnate, especially with chronic inflammatory diseases, exposure to toxic substances or through personal antecedents like unhealthy habits or living conditions.

I've previously mentioned telomeres. Telomeres are a DNA sequence, located at the ends of the chromosomes. They've been studied and written about for several decades now and these studies have established that telomeres are associated with protecting DNA integrity, cellular repair and, consequently, DNA rejuvenation. These findings have revolutionized the subject of cellular regeneration. They've also enriched our understanding of the mechanisms that allow tissues to be repaired. And these are mechanisms integrative medicine has been suggesting for many years.

Many of the recommendations and practices that integrative medicine has associated with cellular regeneration have been around for millennia. Some were inherited from ancestral traditions and are linked to treatment of the energetic field. Yet despite previous clinical evidence to support these practices, the prevailing medical system has mostly ignored them. Fortunately, more recent research, such as the study of telomeres, has demonstrated results with an even more solid basis. This research is now widely acknowledged in the realm of health prevention and regarding physical restoration and repair.

To achieve cellular regeneration, especially when there are imbalances in the mechanisms of renewal, we sometimes need other, stronger stimuli. This is true for instance when the tissues of an organ, apparatus or system have been anatomically and/or functionally altered.

Integrative medicine provides a number of tools whose main objective is to provoke stimuli at the cellular level to support changes in the internal environment. These include changing the pH, increasing oxygenation, decreasing inflammation and improving the absorption and intake of nutrition.

I'll mention here some resources I know particularly well. One is ozone therapy, which is also helpful in the *Remove* phase. It has both a detoxifying and oxygenating effect on the cellular system and supports the process of reparation at that level.

Some other resources I've used are chelation and nutritional and regenerating serum therapies. One in particular is Vitamin C serums, which we use to treat vitamin deficiencies with cancer patients and with others. There are many possible "cocktails" using antioxidant nutrients, selected on a case-by-case basis.

Other interventions include plasma enriched with platelets or platelet growth factors. This is more known for its aesthetic use but it is an excellent aid in the cellular repair of internal organs and also specific tissues, such as joints, in cases of lesions, degenerations and the like.

We also use oral orthomolecular supplemental nutrition in therapeutic doses, to replenish missing or insufficient elements, thus allowing the organism to fully exercise its function.

Energy and body therapies are also invaluable at this stage. Among these, I'll mention acupuncture, *reiki*, biomagnetism and other balance therapies.

In a professional context, these treatments are selected by evaluating the patient with comprehensive diagnostic methods, plus a good clinical history. Personally, I also use an energetic evaluation, microscopic analysis of living cells and a mineralogram scan, which gives us the status of the major minerals in the body and also measures the presence of heavy metals. This is in conjunction with conventional laboratory tests or other clinical or imaging studies, according to the needs of the case.

The repair of cells and tissues generates changes in the symptomatology. By restoring health, we improve an individual's energy level, mood, concentration and overall performance. Protection of the vital organs brings about significant improvements in the quality of life. These changes are especially visible in deteriorating states, long-evolving degenerative diseases or metabolic diseases that are still partly or totally reversible.

At this stage, the detoxification system itself is fortified, collaborating with digestive processes, creating a positive circuit of influence throughout the system. In people who are medicated, the dose of medication can sometimes be considerably reduced. Sometimes it's even possible to suspend the dosage, under medical supervision. *Repair* is a stage where many symptoms subside. In fact, many patients leave treatment at this point, even if they haven't completed the process, because they feel cured. In our culture, the disappearance of symptoms is synonymous with resolution.

In short, much can be achieved at this time. But though I've mentioned various therapies, the most important work is still yours: your daily practices, caring for yourself with the measures I'm suggesting and following the path to better your quality of life.

On the emotional level, *Repair* has to do with reconciling deep wounds and mechanisms that were established some time ago, particularly in childhood, and which cause a kind of noise. *Repair* also has to do with education in emotional intelligence and learning tools to manage and process feelings more from the healthy and empowered adult.

At the same time, it's a job of inclusion and restoration of balance at all possible levels. This phase tunes the personal *antennae*. It gives us better access to the inner wisdom we all have, once we're able to recognize our beliefs, our programs, our unconscious decrees and emotional tapes. Then as we grow stronger, we begin to take other steps for themselves. We open the way to the next phase.

As I've said, in the early stages of emotional management, we re-examine our history, beginning the conscious release of emotional toxins. As our story is understood, released and repaired, we begin to manage our emotions better. And though I'm articulating this process separately as a way to understand it, much of this comes together on its own. Sometimes even just by bringing things to light the regenerative movement has already begun.

The process of reparation also sometimes reveals things we didn't previously realize. This information, which amplifies our history, comes from our *internal images*, which are unconscious familial or personal patterns. It emerges from what we've jealously guarded or hidden in order to survive. Sometimes, as these things emerge, the movement toward change is catalyzed.

The *Repair* phase is when we recognize and reaffirm our story and make reconnections. It's a time to link our symptom or whatever moved us to seek help with our limiting beliefs, conversations and internal dialogues that were buried. It's a recognition from experience, not from intellect. It arises from reconnecting with pain, with our root causes, and giving them a conscious direction or channel. The body is the perfect partner here, as it's often a matter of understanding why we've gotten a disease and then connecting with that through the "body of pain."

In addition to the physical work, *Repair* is the art of curing, closing, completing and relieving emotional pain. From there we set forth with new codes, new answers and a new approach. When we change our perception, our emotional responses change. We begin to rewrite our history as a healthier, more conscious and more life-affirming adult.

CHAPTER 22

TELOMERES: LIVE LONGER AND BETTER

"Aging and dying are normal and expected parts of one's life, we cannot change it. What can change is the way we live until the last day that touches us, including our biological conditions, our health, vitality and joy."

— RAQUELINA LUNA

Epigenetics is the study of changes in the activity of genes that, instead of DNA mutations, are transmitted through cell divisions and multiple generations.[29] Throughout our lives, the epigenome records the experiences of the cell, including developmental changes, environmental influences and its general state of health. In other words, epigenetic mechanisms leave marks that act like memory for cells. So our lifestyle, level of stress and our whole relationship with our environment influences our biology.[30] This is the direct link between our habits and the internal biological world at the cellular level.

But the epigenome is not static; it can be modified, which means these changes are reversible. We can activate and deactivate the expression of genes according to our behavior.

Researchers like Bruce Lipton have shared their visionary perspective on the question of how we can create a cell environment to influence and benefit our cellular interior.[31] Biologist Nathalie Zammatteo previously devoted herself to this research and now works directly with people applying these notions. She has championed the concept that our actions and reactions permanently shape the expression of our genes.[32]

This all sounds cutting edge, but in fairness most of these ideas are very old, especially those related to lifestyle. Ancient traditions such as in China linked specific health systems and therapeutic methods and proposed many of the same things.

As early as the 1930s, Paul Hermann Müller (1948 Nobel Prize winner) and Barbara McClintock (1983 Nobel Prize winner) observed the structures at the ends of the chromosomes, the telomeres. But in recent years, there have been new scientific contributions which demonstrate a direct relationship between telomeres and the enzyme telomerase relating to the health of tissues. For these contributions, Elizabeth Blackburn, Carol Greider and Jack Szostak were awarded the 2009 Nobel Prize in Medicine and are now considered the "parents" of telomerase.

The discoveries of Blackburn, Greider and Szostak added a new and important dimension to our understanding of the cell, explaining the protective function of telomeres and deepening our knowledge of telomerase, the enzyme responsible for their elongation.[33] All of this has shed light on the mechanisms of certain diseases and stimulated the development of potential new therapies.

Long telomeres are directly proportional to greater health, the possibility of slowing cellular aging and a longer life. So the telomeres themselves indicate how our health can be improved and our lives extended. This discovery offers great hope for people with unfortunate genetic conditions or deterioration.

As a special part of DNA situated at the ends of the chromosomes, the role of telomeres is to protect cellular integrity. In each cell division, all genetic material is doubled, so that each new cell creates a nearly perfect copy. But each division comes at a price, because the ends of the telomeres are slightly shortened. It's as if you photocopied a document over and over and each time the last letter of each line was left off. Eventually, the document would make no sense. And eventually, when the lengths of the telomeres are reduced to a significant degree, the cells can no longer replicate and they die or become senescent. This interferes with the correct functioning of the organ to which they belong, causing deterioration and disease.

Our genetics influence our telomeres as to their length at our birth and the speed with which they shorten. And of course, this shortening is also a consequence of cell division and aging and is responsible for accelerating disease (as opposed to elongation, which forestalls it). But the process can be retarded by the enzyme telomerase, which keeps telomeres in good condition and can even regenerate their length to some degree, allowing for additional cell divisions and slightly delaying the cell clock. As Elizabeth Blackburn has said, if we take care of our telomeres, we can live not only a longer life but a better one.[34]

In 2008, Evadnie Rampersaud, professor of genetic epidemiology at the University of Miami, published a study documenting the absence of obesity in Pennsylvania's Amish community, despite the fact that many Amish are carriers of a genetic predisposition for obesity. Rampersaud demonstrated that this genetic predisposition is disabled by the constant physical exercise of these individuals, who by the precepts of their religion are forbidden to use motor vehicles and machines.[35]

"When we take a stroll or go out walking, we don't just burn calories, we also modify the activity of the genes in the hypothalamus and deactivate the effect of the one that opens our appetite," says Jörg Blench, biologist, biochemist and author of the book, *Fate is Not Written in the Genes*.[36]

Blackburn also asserts that we're born with a certain set of genes but our way of living can condition the way these genes are expressed. In some cases, lifestyle factors can turn them on or off.[37]

Clearly, aging doesn't progress linearly toward disease and deterioration. Cellular aging is a dynamic process that can accelerate or slow down and in many cases, damage can be reversed. We are all going to age but how that unfolds will largely depend on our cellular health, because our cells don't simply fulfill the orders of our genetic code.

The food we eat, physical exercise, our reactions to emotional challenges, our sense of security, our environmental quality, even the exposure to stress from intrauterine life or infancy; all are important influences on telomeres.

It's a comforting rebuttal to the certainty that genes fully determine our destiny. This of course doesn't deny the influence of our genes, but we are closer now to a balance of seeing nature and nurture as going hand in hand. George Bray, an endocrinologist and researcher at the University of Louisiana, says it like this, "Genes carry the weapon and the environment pulls the trigger."[38]

To focus on the cellular level is a different way of looking at health, but it's not just for scientists. It's for you, for me, for everyone. The good news is that studies have shown that lifestyle changes can increase telomerase and telomere length within a period of three weeks to four months.

Here are some factors that have been proven to influence the length of your telomeres and promote their elongation.

NUTRITION AND LONG TELOMERES

Healthy foods not only provide nutrients and fuel for all of the organs in your body, they also help you maintain an ideal weight. And as multiple studies have shown, maintaining optimal weight can add years to your life.

One of the best ways to care for telomeres is through diet, so it's recommended that we avoid the regular excess of red meats, sugar and processed food (bread, white rice, pasta, cookies). Beneficial foods include fresh fruits and vegetables, whole grain cereals, legumes, fish and seafood, olive oil, nuts and spices.

Studies have shown that this type of diet prevents cardiovascular disease and heart attacks, metabolic syndrome, dementia and other imbalances. Also, rather than reducing fats, we need to consider what kind of fats we consume. Along with carbohydrates, fats are one of the main sources of energy in our body, which makes them essential to our diet. The so-called unsaturated fats found in vegetables (and in seeds, coconut, avocado, nuts), fish and other foods are necessary for the proper functioning of our organism.

Green leafy vegetables such as spinach, kale, turnip leaves and romaine lettuce are the best sources of lutein and zeaxanthin, folic acid and antioxidants such as beta carotenes, Vitamin C, and Vitamin K1. In general, naturally grown plants are also rich in solar energy in the form of tiny particles of light called biophotons. Sunlight is vital to life and you can absorb this solar energy through the food you eat, as well as through the skin. A high-powered vegetable is broccoli, rich in antioxidants and a lot of isothiocyanates. Other important vegetables include watercress, arugula and radish. Research shows that eating cruciferous vegetables can significantly reduce the risk of breast, bladder, prostate, and lung cancer.

Whenever possible, buy organic vegetables. Organic plants have been shown to have a higher nutritional content than fresh vegetables grown with chemicals. Likewise, eating organic foods we avoid the extra damage caused by chemical fertilizers and pesticides.

Blackberries or blueberries are a great source of nutrition, leading the list of vegetables and fruits. They're very rich in antioxidants that help your body neutralize free radicals (molecules that can cause cell damage). They fight oxidative stress and have a special effect on brain cells. Chlorella is a single cell freshwater algae and is considered a super food. It plays a very important role in the body's disposal of heavy metals, especially mercury.

When garlic is crushed or chopped it produces the compound allicin, which causes the strong smell and taste we all know. It's actually an extremely effective antioxidant. When it's digested in the body, allicin produces sulfonic acid, a compound that reacts quickly with free radicals, faster than any other known compound.

Optimizing insulin levels is also essential for cell anti-aging. You can achieve this by eliminating or reducing your consumption of grains and sugars. Along with the inclusion of natural anti-aging foods, this is an extremely crucial step for improved health and longevity.

Although we actually need a balance of a wide variety of nutrients, some more specific recommendations are worth mentioning. This is because many people lack many of these important ingredients and there's scientific confirmation of those benefits. Following the suggestions of Dr. Blackburn, I'll mention these anti-aging nutrients: astaxanthin, coenzyme Q-10, Vitamin D, omega 3, magnesium, Vitamin K2, polyphenols (mainly found in grapes, cocoa, green tea) and probiotics.[39] Also Vitamin B12, folic acid and curcumin (found in turmeric).

MORE SUGGESTIONS FOR YOUR TELOMERES

Intermittent fasting

As previously explained, this consists of scheduling meals in order to allow regular periods of fasting. Professor Cynthia Kenyon, an American geneticist specializing in cellular aging, has shown that reducing carbohydrates, as one does with intermittent fasting, activates genes that determine youth and longevity.[40] It's important to remember that with this kind of fasting you also need to decrease sugars and maintain quality in food.

Regular physical exercise

It's also vital to have a complete exercise program. This is another lifestyle factor that will radically improve the sensitivity of insulin receptors.

High-intensity exercise decreases the aging process by naturally reducing the shortening of telomeres. In fact, there's a direct association between a decrease in the shortening of telomeres and high intensity exercise. The only caveat is that we must avoid overtraining to the point of extreme fatigue and muscle damage, because this can also damage the functions by which we repair and the recovery is taxing.

Deep sleep and rest

Sleep deprivation and going through the day on only a few hours of rest have been associated with DNA damage that decreases telomere length and causes cellular aging. This affects not only adults, but also children, and it has long-term consequences. This discovery was outlined in a study from Princeton University published by the *Journal of Pediatrics*.[41]

Stress management

Prolonged stress has also been associated with shorter telomeres. It's been discovered that extreme emotions, a charged mental state and responses to stressful demands have a significant impact on telomeres.

The negative effects of stress begin before conception. The pre-existing physical health of the mother makes up the

intrauterine environment of a baby. The work of Sonja En-
tringer, Pathik Wadhwa and others has demonstrated that
the greater the prenatal anxiety of a mother, the shorter the
telomere length of the baby. This sets the stage for an accelerated path of aging.[42]

The transgenerational transmission of risks should also
be taken into account, as should early adversities such as
severe neglect and abuse.

I'll discuss stress further in Chapter 29, but it's clear
that at any stage of life we should avoid or manage chronic
stress and fatigue and learn to deal with stressful situations
as challenges rather than simply as threats. These are important steps to improve or maintain telomeric length.

I invite you once again to set forth on a R.E.A.L. path toward optimal health. Start by avoiding actions you already
know aren't good for you. At the same time, begin to incorporate other simple practices and observe how they work in
you. Experiment with yourself. Give yourself time to notice
the benefits and make a habit of doing what's best for you.

Make the changes that are in your power. You can start
to live better and more fully. Now, right now.

ACTIONS FOR A R.E.A.L. LIFE

Check your pantry and your grocery list. Start to include healthier and more suitable meals for you.

Get involved in preparing your food. Explore new ingredients and new recipes.

Make your exercise plan. Start moving today. You don't have to wait until Monday or the beginning of next month. Identify something you enjoy so you can stick with it and not feel it as imposition. Make moving fun. Explore options.

Incorporate 30 minutes daily of meditation or mindfulness.

Discover your pattern of responding to stress and find solutions that work better for you.

Get to bed earlier to guarantee more and deeper sleep.

CHAPTER 23

THE ART OF EATING WELL

"May your food be your medicine."

– HIPPOCRATES

Food and nutrition make up the physical foundation on which the general balance of the body rests. To compare it with nature, the body is the earth from which all things can grow if they have adequate fertilizer, water, light, cleansing and care. Food supplies the body with the nutrients and energy it needs to stay healthy. For the diet to be balanced, the necessary quality, variety and quantity of nutrients will vary according to the person's age, bodily constitution, physical condition, the geography, activities and so on.

I know it can be confusing to choose what diet is best as there are so many different opinions out there. My intent here is not to provide you with the *truth*, but rather to simply share some suggestions from my studies, my research and my own experience. Nor will I go into very specific aspects on the subject of nutrition; that could be a whole separate book. My goal is to introduce the topic in a practical way with a general approach that emphasizes what's vital for the organism to regenerate and to maintain the best possible balance. Because no matter what trend you follow, there are general aspects of nutrition that are valid and applicable in almost every case. Food is essential for life, a fundamental pillar of health. Of all the habits which determine the renewal and longevity of the human being, nutrition has been studied the most. Nutrition is directly related to the appearance of cardiovascular and metabolic diseases, among many others. Eating well, in a varied and complete way, allows our body to function normally, covering basic biological needs. At the same time, it also prevents or reduces the risk of short and long-term illness or imbalance.

It's worth considering the impact in our times of so-called "diseases of civilization," like diabetes, hypertension, obesity, cardiovascular diseases, eating disorders and even certain types of cancer that relate to diet. There isn't always a direct cause-effect relationship, but diet is an important factor that can add to a greater risk of the onset and development of these diseases.

In recent years, research has yielded both interesting and important data linking the human microbiota to many of the health imbalances I've just mentioned. You may not know this, but there's a living, microscopic world in your intestines called intestinal microbiota or gut flora. With about 100 billion bacteria, the microbial ecosystem of the intestine consists of many native species that permanently colonize the gastrointestinal tract as well as a variable series of microorganisms that only do so transitively. Experts now consider this community of micro-organisms, their genes and their metabolites as a "new organ" whose specific functions are key to maintaining our good health.

Collectively, the microbiota are responsible for two vital functions: helping to regulate the energy supply and protecting us from invaders (viruses, fungi and disease-generating bacteria). They are influenced, however, by external factors, including birth conditions, diet, the environment or use of antibiotics. Intestinal microbiota disorders have been associated with conditions as dissimilar as asthma, chronic inflammatory diseases, immunological diseases, obesity and non-alcoholic steatohepatitis. The composition of the microbiota has also been linked to the risk of psychiatric and neurodegenerative diseases such as depression and Alzheimer's, although this research is still in process.

Dr. Thomas Rau emphasizes that 80% of an adult's immune defenses reside in the small intestine and that in children the percentage may be even higher.[43] In addition, more than 100 million brain-connected neurons live in the intestine. In other words, our defenses, the relative resistance or vulnerability of our body, and the overall quality of our health are greatly linked to our nutrition.

This issue of food is a real challenge. We are bombarded with tantalizing invitations to consume foods with high caloric content, processed sugars, additives, preservatives and on and on. These are foods that are appetizing and attractive to olfactory nerves and palates that are used to them, but they attack the microbiota and influence the shortening of telomeres.

These days, instead of our food being a preventative tool or one of our health maintenance resources, it's unfortunately the opposite. It's very difficult for people to really accept this notion. Sometimes they only do so because a significant health concern compels them. For many, to eat healthily and well is not a pleasant experience. It's something they suffer through to get healthier but they see it as a temporary parenthesis in their lives.

Most people eat what they have, what they like, what fills the stomach or satiates the appetite. It doesn't matter what they eat or how much. And if they combine that unconscious diet with a high level of stress, lack of rest and a sedentary routine – not to mention other physical and emotional variables – there's a perfect recipe for the deterioration of the body and a diminishment of its ability to self-balance. Among many other consequences, we get the accumulation of fat, excess weight, blocked arteries, the vascular endothelium is damaged, the general system starts to decline and lose control and its ability to cope with internal changes diminishes. This triggers multiple possibilities for disease, depending on individual predispositions and the type of excess or imbalance.

The vital fuel the body uses as energy for survival comes from our food. That's why food is the foundation for providing the basic energy for all the other processes of change. With more energy and a more balanced body you can focus on other aspects. You can work on your emotions and dedicate yourself to a healthier and more expansive spiritual practice. A real change, beyond the subtle levels of the soul, definitely requires work with the body. And the first step is diet.

Eating well is an art. To introduce yourself to that art, besides being interested in knowing a bit more, you need to create a consciousness and above all a connection with your body to stimulate the inspiration to keep that temple in peak condition. Remember, everything that will happen to you is made possible by your body.

The diet a person is exposed to while growing up and the habits that were established at home are hugely influential. So developing the art of eating well requires going beyond the pleasures your palate may be used to, and avoiding all the delicious, less healthy options, which are everywhere.

The art of eating well invites you to get involved in the selection and the processing of the foods you bring to your table and share with those you love. I suggest that you discover in other foods, flavors and ways of cooking a new palate through which you connect with your mind and heart, because eating with consciousness is an act of love.

Reconnecting with the sublime pleasure of eating will help you to end the war with food and with the obsessive craving that comes with extreme dietary limitations or with the complete lack of control which indulges anything.

To make the transition and help manage the temptations, stock up on what's best for you. You eat more of what you have on hand, so reduce the consumption of junk food by not having it readily available. This kind of decision helps a lot. Likewise, if you have healthier food on hand, the chances of eating it greatly increase. That's a good way to start changing personal and family habits.

I'll share some suggestions for you to initiate the change or to reaffirm it. At the same time, I invite you to continue the investigation. You can definitely have a huge impact on your transformation, maybe more than you think. You have power over your health, over the direction you give your life, over your happiness. To quote the poet William Ernest Henley, you can truly be "the master of your fate" and "the captain of your soul."

To eat consciosly is an act of love.

ACTIONS FOR A R.E.A.L. LIFE

Experiment with varied flavors, add new ingredients; increase the range that your palate considers pleasant. Dare to taste new foods, new flavors.

Don't fill yourself to the extreme. Stop when you feel satisfied, even if you have more space. One way to support yourself in this is to serve yourself small portions.

From time to time, get your children to participate in the preparation of food. It's an excellent way for kids to agree to try new foods.

Practicing mindfulness will help you enjoy your food and control the amount you eat.

Avoid canned, processed foods and food with preservatives. Avoid artificial dyes and flavorings. Avoid temperature extremes in your meals. Eat less sugar.

Reduce the total amount of fat you consume by eliminating fried foods, saturated fats and sources of trans-fatty acids, such as butter, margarine, solidified butter, hydrogenated oils.

Even if you're not a vegetarian, make vegetables the basis of your food in a variety of ways.

Increase your consumption of omega-3 fatty acids by eating fish containing them, as well as flax oil, linseed seeds, chia seeds, quinoa, nuts.

Minimize your consumption of processed meat and derived products such as sausages and whole dairy products. They are related to cancer and other diseases. Develop a preference for organic, natural and pesticide-free products that do not harm your body.

Set your schedule by your dietary plan and respect it.

These are just a few suggestions. I invite you to continue the research. Find out, amplify your options.

CHAPTER 24

SUGAR!

*"There is a country in the world placed in an unlikely
archipelago of sugar and alcohol . . ."*

— PEDRO MIR

I dedicate this chapter to all my diabetic ancestors and especially my father who, as a "good family member," was also diabetic. He was one of many who suffered and died from the complications of this disease. I address my loving and inclusive gaze to all those who didn't survive or couldn't recover their health because of diabetes.

Diabetes isn't the only disease directly related to high sugar consumption and the body's inability to handle it. New discoveries are being made all the time concerning the harm excess sugar causes in the body, including the predisposition to cancer.

One could say that sugar as a general flavor is the predominate favorite of the Western palate. The typical Western diet is heavily loaded with sweet, either because it's added on purpose or because, as in many pre-prepared foods, it's masked. In my country of origin, the Dominican Republic, when you drink something sweet it's very sweet. Even coffee, whose bitter taste makes it special, is sweetened with lots of sugar by most Dominicans to make it *rico*.

Our sugar consumption is so high that we completely take it for granted. When offered a juice or coffee you're rarely asked if you want sugar; they simply add it in advance. On top of all that, in our imitation of foreign cultures, we adopt foods and processes typical of the United States and loaded with sugar.

Obesity, diabetes, metabolic syndrome and cancer are "diseases of civilization" associated with the indiscriminate consumption of sugars, especially refined sugar. It's one of the agents that most contribute to the damage of intestinal microbiota. Due to the inflammation levels, endothelial damage, mineral imbalance, lipid profile alteration and other internal damage caused by sugar, it's also associated with inflammatory, degenerative and autoimmune diseases such as arthritis, asthma, multiple sclerosis, arteriosclerosis and cardiovascular disease. Additionally, sugar causes a rapid rise in adrenaline, hyperactivity and anxiety, which in children causes difficulty concentrating and irritability.

The abuse of sugar can also cause problems with the gastrointestinal tract, such as heartburn, indigestion, poor absorption in patients with intestinal problems, increased risk of Crohn's disease and ulcerative colitis. It's one of the triggers of these increasingly prevalent diseases, including among young people. Also, not surprisingly, sugar is associated with premature aging.

Statistics collected in the Dominican Republic from a 2017 study by the National Diabetes Institute and the Ibero-American University show that more than one million Dominicans suffer from diabetes, which was at the time about 13% of the population. Other studies indicate that the number of those affected by the "sickness of sweet" may be closer to 15%. It's also worth noting that 58% of diabetics also suffer from hypertension. This is true not only in the Dominican Republic but throughout Latin America, although the world's highest percentages are found in the

Caribbean. However, the Pan American Health Organization has said that due to an alarming increase in recent years, diabetes is approaching epidemic proportions. Globally, the WHO estimates that more than 346 million people have diabetes and if the current trend continues, this number will likely double by 2030.

Statistics also show that the number of overweight or obese people of all ages is increasing. In the United States, between 7% and 12% of children under the age of five are obese. For adolescents the number is one in five. For adults the rate of those obese or overweight is close to 60%. And of course these figures are expected to increase if we continue down the same road.

It is definitely important to know more about the issue, especially since sugar is an additive in most processed foods. People don't notice it but this contributes to its addictive power. Added sugar, under various forms and names, is an ingredient in more foods than we suspect. I've actually made a list with 99 different names used for sugar (see Appendix II). Here are some the most common: corn syrup, cane syrup, maple syrup, honey, molasses, lactose, maltose, sucrose, dextrose, fructose and concentrated fruit juice. You might also be surprised at the high concentration of sugar in some foods, such as barbecue sauces (BBQ), ketchup, dressings, milk, yogurt, cereals, energy bars, chicken and other charcoal or grill products, various flavorings, etc. It's important also to add that rice, pasta and bread (especially refined breads) have a high sugar content. Whole wheat cereals are better options because they have fibers, but they should still be consumed moderately.

Some research suggests that sugar addiction can act in the brain in the same way as substances like tobacco and even cocaine. In 2007, after a series of tests comparing sugar with cocaine, researchers at the University of Bordeaux came to the conclusion that intense sweetness can exceed the sense of "reward" produced by cocaine, even in drug-sensitized individuals.[44] It's believed that this addictive potential is caused by an innate hypersensitivity in the brain to sweet taste stimulants, awakening a stronger sensation than is possible with cocaine. Given all of this, you can see why it's so hard to stop consuming sugar. It also serves to discredit the explanations of sudden cravings for sugar as a product of low blood sugar, as opposed to being an addictive response.

It's worth noting that the WHO recommends that we consume a maximum of 25 grams of sugar per day. That's less than is found in a single soda or a glass of orange juice. I'm alarmed just thinking about our children's snacks at school. That would be an excellent place to make changes; once of course we adults have begun to make ours.

Remember, even if you're thin, it doesn't mean you can eat whatever you want because you don't get fat. Weight is important but health is not just a matter of weight. Thin people also have to take care in what they eat. They should take the same precautions as overweight people and also exercise.

As for having a plan to change your dietary habits and sticking to it, try to get others excited in your workplace, at home or in the family. This improves the experience and makes it easier to bear.

Since sugar is addictive, once you decide to reduce your consumption to the recommended level, prepare yourself mentally to feel the craving and to handle it well. Put yourself in a positive frame of mind. Identify with the process as a gift you're giving yourself. You're choosing to take care of yourself. Visualize yourself looking healthier, with more vitality and joy. If it still gives you a lot of anxiety, try a vegetable first or fruit. Try to distract yourself. Do a favorite activity. After the critical period has passed, in 48- 72 hours, the anxiety will begin to decrease. You'll begin to feel better, less anxious with more energy and even mental clarity. You'll be leaving behind a dependence that's been correlated with fatigue, depression, anxiety, poor sleep habits and hormonal and digestive problems.

Along with what you're able to do for yourself, your best prize will be discovering your inner strength in this and other aspects of your health. You will grow in personal power, in respect and in self-love. Stay with the belief that you can change your habits to gain quality of life. And if you already have any of the various diseases linked to health habits, you can always improve and reach the optimal level possible.

It's not necessary to eliminate all sugar, because we definitely need the caloric intake of carbohydrates to work. Instead, it's about being aware how many sources we take it from and learning to calculate it. I admit it's a bit of an awkward task at first. It's difficult in our culture to find low sugar or zero sugar products. But I'll share some ideas below that might be useful.

ACTIONS FOR A R.E.A.L. LIFE

Start by not adding sugar to juices, smoothies, chips, cereals and everything you prepare.

Learn to read labels and observe the nutritional value of the packaged foods you buy. Discover the sugar content of the unprocessed and natural products you eat and consider healthy and that you sometimes consume without measure, such as fruits.

Learn the other names so you can recognize sugar sources that are masked (see Appendix II).

Try to count and consciously record the grams of sugar you take in daily, and reduce its consumption to a healthy amount.

Consume carbohydrates in moderation, such as rice, pasta, potatoes and roots. Be careful with products that say light diet, lite, low carb or low fat. Many of them also contain sugar and many people consume these in large quantities since they're considered dietary products.

CHAPTER 25

DΣΣP RΣST

"Sweet Rest not only invigorates the body, but also the spirit."
— OVID

Many people don't know how to disconnect and rest. Even if they sleep a lot they don't get quality sleep. Many others just don't sleep enough. Learning to rest is essential to maintain health, especially when you're in a healing process and entering the phase of *Repair*.

To rest means periodically stopping during the day and doing nothing for a while. You can sit and breathe or lie down for a few minutes to relax the body, or take a nap or simply contemplate the horizon for a bit. Learning to rest also definitely means getting enough sleep at night at a deep enough level of sleep.

Rest, like sleep, is part of our biological rhythms and improves our quality of life. Without it, our mental concentration and physical performance are diminished, while at the same time our nervous system is more irritable. Prolonged lack of rest can lead to slower thinking and slower reactions. It can diminish your capacity to deal with stressful situations and solve problems. It can lead to progressive mental disorders and energetic and physical exhaustion.

Maybe you've already experienced some of these things.

Rest means you enter a low state of mental and physical activity, which allows you to be refreshed and ready to continue your daily activities. It's not just inactivity. It requires tranquility, relaxation and release from anxiety.

The mechanisms of self-regulation and self-repair, together with the biological cycles and natural, intelligent processes of our organism, are empowered and optimized with the right environment and sufficient body energy. And among the most important factors for generating this energy are rest and deep sleep.

Conscious restfulness stimulates healing and you support this process by reaching a state in which the parasympathetic nervous system begins to initiate action. The parasympathetic nervous system relaxes the body and inhibits many vital functions. As Dr. Hamer has explained, an illness often becomes more uncomfortable at night, with more pronounced symptoms, because as we rest the repair mechanisms are actively engaged with the illness.[45]

During sleep, at night, we have less activity of the brain, heart and respiratory system. It's estimated that during sleep, 75% of our growth hormone is secreted. This hormone plays a key role in the repair and regeneration of muscle tissue and bones and also influences the burning of body fat as fuel.

Sleep is a state of altered consciousness whose primary function is to restore your energy and well-being. It is characterized by a minimum of physical activity, variable levels of consciousness, changes in the body's physiological processes and decreased response to external stimuli. The biological processes that occur during sleep are complex and depend on a variety of neurochemicals in the central nervous system and changes in the peripheral nervous system, the cardiovascular, respiratory, endocrine and muscle systems, and others.

The human body is naturally governed by an internal biological clock that dictates when to wake and when to sleep. This cycle is called the circadian rhythm. All basic biological rhythms are programmed on the basis of the solar rhythm. Darkness is in fact what stimulates melatonin, a hormone secreted by the pineal gland that's responsible for regulating our biological clock, among other things. It makes us aware of time and its cycles. The melatonin increases in the evening and induces us to sleep. In the morning it decreases and it's easier to wake up.

Poor sleep quality can weaken your immune system and predispose you to heart disease, stomach ulcers, mood disorders, depression and other consequences. In persons with a predisposition, it can collaborate with pre-diabetic states, metabolic syndrome and weight gain. In the case of tumors, it can contribute to an acceleration of their growth.

Not sleeping seriously affects your memory even after just one night; it impacts your ability to think clearly the next day. Sleep restores normal levels of brain activity and the balance between different parts of the nervous system. It also restores the natural balance between the neural centers. In the long run, sleep deprivation induces premature aging by interfering with the production of growth hormone, which is mostly released during sleep, by the pituitary gland.

There are many possible physical causes for insomnia or poor quality sleep, including a melatonin deficiency, prolonged use of certain pharmaceuticals or drugs, nocturia (a frequent need to urinate at night), an excess of caffeine and certain endocrine disorders. There are also important ambient or environmental variables to consider, such as: the quality of the mattress, ventilation, lighting, smells, noise or the presence of additional lights (e.g. digital lights on a watch or electrical equipment such as a TV).

Sleeplessness can also be caused by a specific anxiety, emotional or mental blockages, tensions or accumulated worries that translate into insecurity and fear. These can then trigger other mechanisms which keep a person alert and unwilling to lose control.

In the systemic approach, insomnia is interpreted as a conscious or unconscious need to stay watchful. From this point of view, an unconscious insomnia could be associated with unresolved conflicts from the past that have been passed down transgenerationally. These conflicts might be the traumatic or unexpected death of a family member or any unexplained loss or the deaths of family members who couldn't be mourned at the time.

The amount of hours a person should sleep is a matter of diverse opinions. The truth is that it's variable and can be different for each person. There are a small number of people who only need between five and six hours a night. Others, however, may require 10 hours or more. For a healthy adult, the WHO recommends an average of seven to eight hours.

The sleep cycle is composed of five phases. The third and fourth are those of deep sleep, the most restorative and most directly related to metabolic and hormonal changes. It is in these phases of sleep that the brain uses less glucose, the pituitary gland segregates less corticosteroids and the nervous and muscular systems are less active, so insulin levels are regulated. This is because the body needs less energy and glucose metabolism decreases.

When you sleep less than six hours or when the quality of your sleep is poor, your health deteriorates. When your health is already deteriorated and you need to recover it, the lack of sleep costs you a lot more.

ACTIONS FOR A R.E.A.L. LIFE

If you need to improve your sleep and rest, try these suggestions:

Identify the emotional, environmental or nutritional factors that alter your sleep quality. Learn to avoid things that promote insomnia.

Darken your bedroom: block light from windows as well as your cellphone or any electrical equipment. If necessary, get a sleep mask to wear over years.

Decrease electromagnetic pollution by leaving your cellphone outside the room or turning it off. Turn off your Wi-Fi router when you sleep. Remove electrical devices (like a TV) from the room. You should reserve your bedroom for sleep and relaxation, instead of work or watching TV.

Take a walk about two hours for bedtime.

Prepare yourself mentally for about an hour before you go to bed. Stop working and start relaxing. Send messages to yourself about your readiness to sleep. Listen to soothing music, write in a diary or read something uplifting.

Set up a bedtime routine. This might include a warm shower or bath, meditation, prayer or deep breathing. You might use aromatherapy or essential oils (e.g. lavender, chamomile, cypress, jasmine, sandalwood). Self-massage could help, or a massage from your partner. Put a cotton swab of essential lavender oil under your pillow, or apply the oil to your body after bathing.

Try flower therapy or flower essences, which are natural and have no side effects. A formula designed specifically for you might be helpful.

Get a weekly massage or some other body therapy to loosen your muscles.

Listen to relaxation tapes, guided visualizations or practice mindfulness sleep exercises.

Avoid eating full meals before bedtime, especially fattening foods or with lots of sugar.

Go to bed earlier. Your adrenal system recharges most of its energy between 11:00 p.m. and 1:00 a.m.

General measures: exercise regularly, minimize caffeine and alcohol, eat healthier and maintain a healthy weight. And if you need it: seek physical, emotional or psychological help to identify other possible obstacles to deep sleep and rest.

ACTIONS FOR CHILDREN

Most of the above measures also apply to children. It also helps them during their first few years to lie in bed with them for a while. If they have difficulty sleeping and they have some bonding issue or significant fears, you can lie in bed with them with the additional intention of re-establishing their sense of safety and trust. Hug them from behind so they fall asleep feeling protected. In this way, they can let go of their deeper stress responses and their psyche can heal.

In my book for children, *Los Colores del Amor (The Colors of Love)*, there's a guided visualization on the accompanying CD that's specifically for bedtime. It's not available in English at present, but you can often find useful visualizations online.

If all of this isn't enough, get help. Your child may need special therapeutic aids such as acupuncture, *reiki*, breathing techniques, nutritional supplements, psychological or even psychiatric help. In any case, always consult your pediatrician.

CHAPTER 26

MY EXPERIENCE WITH CANCER

"Through sickness, Life tells us," I'm still giving you a chance."

— RAQUELINA LUNA

I'm going to elaborate on my experience of having cancer. I feel I've been blessed with the opportunity to keep living and I want to share the experience as a support to others. After telling the story, I'll briefly mention the more important treatments I used, before and after my surgery. Many are part of the repertoire of therapies I've used for a long time in treating patients with cancer, as well other diseases or imbalances.

According to the American Thyroid Association, medullary thyroid carcinoma makes up just 1-2% of thyroid cancers and usually metastasizes quickly to lymph nodes and other organs. Medullary thyroid cancer is considered one of the more aggressive types of cancer, with a generally less positive prognosis than many and only a few conventional treatment options. Depending on the stage of the disease, it can be treated with surgery, radiation or chemotherapy.

Despite the many advances in science and the fact that we all know having cancer is not necessarily a death sentence, receiving that kind of diagnosis is one of those moments that truly confronts a person. It certainly confronted me. The fact is, we never expect something like that. We never think it will happen to us. When my doctor gave me the diagnosis, his words echoed in my head for a long time: "It's cancer. You have metastasis and it's very aggressive."

I confess that for several days I was scared to read, to carefully review the results of the biopsy or to look for more medical information. I was afraid to learn more. Hearing that diagnosis sent me through all the emotional phases I'd seen described in books and through other unimaginable ones that simply live in the flesh. My mind leapt to all the threatening, fatal, funereal scenarios and my emotions followed.

I allowed myself to experience the pain and all the reactions that came up. I didn't deny, avoid or ignore them. Instead, I let them pass through my body. I gave myself the permission to live with all of them and I became that "body of pain." At that point, they were my teachers. I cried, shouted and felt in every pore that mixture of anguish, indignation, anger, deep sadness, abandonment and even guilt. I questioned my life, my beliefs and my work. It was the strongest confrontation I've ever experienced but I accepted it. This helped me pass through the arc of emotions and reach the other polarity where the confidence, serenity and love began to appear. Little by little, the calm arrived and I came back to the center and the connection with my inner resilience. I reorganized my ideas and emotions. This time had to be "about me." I had to take charge and so I did. Cancer had brought me to the edge of a precipice facing death, so I could look at life.

I realized something obvious that we take for granted: I was alive. Cancer invited me to see it. And it told me more: "If you're alive, you have options." My heart began to embrace cancer and accept what was happening. Because to accept it was to let go of questioning and judgment and to look equally at life and death. I wanted to live, yes, and at the same time I was humbly surrendering to a greater plan. I found peace in living one day at a time, only now, only today. I appreciated every sunrise, every breath, the warm shower, the clean sheets, the supplements I was taking, the hands that touched me, every resource and every kind of help that came to me. The colors, the flavors, the views, the silences, the mountains, the hugs, having hot tea, the clouds, everything seemed like a miracle.

With that attitude and with gratitude toward everything, I began my preparation. First, I decided to say yes to the option of surgery. I gave space to both the conventional and the integrative treatments and I welcomed the resources that were already at hand.

I already had a lot of experience treating cancer patients with a complementary approach, which is actually very practical. And curiously, I had just begun to study integrative oncology more formally. So I set to work to prepare as I had learned, to give my body and soul the best opportunity to improve my body's receptivity, to bring my cells to a higher level of vitality and to optimize my general conditions, especially my immune system.

INTEGRATIVE ONCOLOGY

This new specialty within integrative medicine offers cancer patients a series of complementary medical resources based on scientific evidence and in combination with official medicine. It doesn't reject conventional treatments nor does it indiscriminately accept complementary techniques. Integrative oncology has been generally accepted and is now offered by major universities in the United States and Europe. It has also been introduced in several prestigious hospitals, some of which I've had the opportunity to visit.

Integrative oncology was born as an attempt to join conventional medicine (surgery, radiation therapy, chemotherapy, hormone and immunotherapy, etc.) with therapeutic techniques (acupuncture, orthomolecular nutrition, aromatherapy, mindfulness, homeopathy, purification techniques, etc.). The integrative modalities help to strengthen every system in the body, as well as to relieve pain and achieve mental relaxation. This allows the patient to better withstand the adverse effects of conventional protocols and procedures. An integrative approach also treats the patient and their family with individualized treatments, tailored to the patient's needs and preferences. This is achieved with an interdisciplinary team which emphasizes the patient's active role in therapeutic decision-making. Of course, no miraculous cures are promised, but resources are applied that have proven efficacy and can safely be combined with other treatments.

Finally, this approach offers opportunities to those who choose not to conform to an official protocol or who have already exhausted conventional medical options and are looking for other kinds of help.

PREPARATION FOR SURGERY

I set out to "prepare the ground," as I've outlined in the section called *Remove*. I dedicated myself to improving the condition of my body in preparation for my formal treatment: a thyroidectomy and the removal of cervical lymph nodes where the cancer had begun to metastasize.

Anyone can do this kind of preparatory work while seeking opinions or waiting to start a treatment. These measures always do some good. They can be done without a conclusive diagnosis, when there's possible evidence of a catastrophic malignancy or disease or while waiting for the oncologist's recommendations.

"Preparing the ground" is not only meant for cancer and can be applied in any inflammatory process, degenerative or autoimmune disease and various others. In multiple cases I've treated, this phase has caused a great deal of improvement in a patient's symptoms. If there's not much deterioration, there may even be remission. In my case, during this phase the swelling of my cervical nodes dropped significantly until most were no longer perceptible to palpitation. Anyway, it's very advantageous to be in a better condition to receive surgery, chemotherapy, radiation or any other treatment. That was my approach. The organized unification of both integrative and conventional options often brings more promising results.

I had 36 days from the date of my diagnosis to the date for my surgery. I assumed a daily routine that began with meditation, mindfulness exercises and prayer. This helped me feel more relaxed and at peace so I could begin to feel more confident and to let go of judgment and internal struggle. Thankfully, I knew that a calm, less-stressed mental and emotional state improves the internal cellular environment and creates a more empathetic biochemical medium with the immune system.[46]

I put together a selection of music with high vibrations, music that brings me to my center and fills me with sublime feelings. This helped me rest and disconnect from recurring thoughts. When my husband heard how often the same few pieces were repeating, he made me a much more varied and beautiful collection and I often listened to that. I also played music with lyrics I like and I sang with it every day.

I've had a healthy diet for many years now. I've refrained from eating sugar or foods rich in sugar and avoided processed and fried food. I carefully select what I eat. But now I took on a much stricter diet of mostly raw foods. I drank green juices in the morning. I ate a variety of salads, fermented vegetables, some purifying broths, seeds, nuts and some fruits. I also drank turmeric and ginger infusions to which I added a splash of fresh homemade coconut milk. I ate dark chocolate in various ways. I prepared most of my food for myself and my creativity in the kitchen flourished. I respected my sleep hours and slept between eight and nine hours a night. I took naps during the day, which I previously never did. I kept exercising moderately, without exhausting myself. The sport I practice is running, but during this period I took walks or jogged a bit and did simple yoga routines.

I checked everything I apply to my body and began to be more selective with what I used: cosmetics, creams, hair products and so on. I prepared a body oil mixture by combining therapeutic grade essential oils. I applied this topically and also ingested some. I ended up making my own scented spray from all these blends of fragrances.

Every day I did organic coffee enemas. This became a special ritual up to the day before the surgery. Then, 15 days after my surgery, I resumed this practice. I still continue with it, though with less frequency now.

While doing all these preparations, I also reviewed the messages of my subconscious through my body, including my emotions and family systems. I found connections with issues from my childhood. I also took the opportunity to review my emotions during the period when my lymph nodes first became noticeably swollen. This kind of analysis helped me to release even more.

My morning routine was completely dedicated to me. I stayed off of social media and the internet and only used the phone for essential calls. I entered a space-time of greater silence, rest and creative visualizations, many of which I recorded for myself.

With a thankful attitude and "filling my cup of gratitude" every day, I connected with my abundance. And the truth is, I felt fortunate, rich and abundant. Everything I needed came to me. How could I not be thankful? This sense of gratitude helped me take the journey with even more compassion.

When I had thoughts of fear or when I felt myself contracting with uncertainty, I came back to the present. I said to my cancer, "Thank you for keeping me alive." It's not only that I was more serene and in a better place each day, I also felt a great sense of fullness, an appreciation for everything I had.

Another way I stayed mindful of gratitude was to make a literal jar of gratitude and each day I wrote out things I was thankful for on little pieces of paper and put them in the jar. By the day of my surgery, the jar was starting to be full. Thank you!

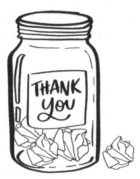

The result of all this preparation, which I did in a relaxed yet focused way, was that I arrived at the surgery room on my own two feet, delivering myself and quietly surrendering to whatever was to be. After the surgery, which was successful, my recovery was very rapid, without pain and without complications. To the astonishment of my doctors at Mount Sinai Hospital in Manhattan, within seven days the tumor markers were already basically normal for my condition, whereas typically they begin to decrease between the first and second month post-surgery. They've remained normal to this day. I haven't needed any additional treatment except to continue my own maintenance plan, which is an anti-cancer life plan that includes the periodic reinforcement of various integrative therapies.

SPECIALIZED TREATMENTS OF INTEGRATIVE MEDICINE

The treatments below are the ones I used to fortify myself. Some of these should be supervised, indicated, and organized in such a manner that they're synergistic with each other and don't create any antagonism with other treatments, such as radiation or chemotherapy. They should be individualized according to each case and condition.

Acupuncture

Acupuncture is one the healing arts of TCM and a 1,000 year-old way of restoring human balance. Acupuncture was my formal introduction to the world of energy medicine and it's a resource that will always have a special place in my heart. The goal of the stimulus is an equilibrium of energy and a restoration of the balance between complementary energies (*yin* and *yang*). Acupuncture has been recognized by the WHO and has spread throughout the West. Nowadays, one can almost count on finding an acupuncturist in most countries. It's also included in the general curriculum of some conventional medical schools and even offered as a major or specialization. In 1997, the FDA reclassified acupuncture as a safe medical resource. They now estimate that Americans make 9 to 12 million visits annually to medical acupuncturists.

Ozone Therapy

Ozone ($O3$) is the triatomic form of oxygen ($O2$) and consists of negative ions. Ozone therapy increases energy levels by increasing the supply of circulating oxygen. In addition, ozone enhances the immune system by improving the activity of T lymphocytes and monocytes charged with releasing cytokines, which are intercellular messengers that can activate the mechanisms of natural immunity. In addition, ozone reduces oxidative stress and reduces inflammation.

By itself, it has not been shown to be an oncologic treatment, but it's helpful in preparing the body and accompanying other treatments. I've been treating patients with ozone therapy for more than 15 years and it's a valuable resource of integral practice.

Vitamin C Serums in Mega-doses

The U.S. National Cancer Institute reports that high intravenous doses of Vitamin C in cancer patients improved their quality of life and decreased the side effects associated with their treatments. It has an antioxidant and also pro-oxidant action on tumor cells, without affecting healthy cells. And when administered by intravenous infusion, Vitamin C can reach higher concentrations in the blood than if the same amount were ingested orally.

At my clinic, Lunavital, we use Vitamin C in high doses to elevate the immune system and to accompany treatments of oncological patients. Since 2008, we've had excellent results supporting patients in preparation for conventional treatments, in recovery afterwards and also in cases where they aren't candidates for any of the classic oncological treatments.

Vitalist Homeopathy

This is an injectable homeopathic product also known as *hansi*. It works in infinitesimal dilutions of various combinations of cactus, aloes and trace elements. This blend of enhanced vegetable and mineral elements stimulates cellular vitality. Its use was initially limited to the treatment of cancer, but it has also proved helpful in treating other diseases, such as AIDS (acquired immunodeficiency syndrome), chronic fatigue syndrome, allergies, multiple sclerosis, rheumatoid arthritis, lupus and viral diseases. *Hansi* acts as a regenerative and stabilizer of the cell membrane and the nutrition inside it.

Mindfulness

Over the past 30 years, the practice of mindfulness has been integrated into Western medicine and psychology. It is recognized as an effective way to reduce stress, increase self-awareness, reduce physical and psychological symptoms associated with stress, and improve overall well-being.

In recent years, studies have been conducted evaluating the mindfulness–based stress reduction program and mindfulness–based cognitive therapy as applied to cancer patients. The results have been promising. For example, a meta-analysis by M. F. Zhang and others found that mindfulness–based therapy was effective in significantly reducing anxiety and depressive symptomatology.[47] Their recommendation of additional research to assess long-term benefits is in process. Many hospitals in the United States and around the world many hospitals are making use of this tool and offering it to cancer patients.

Aromatherapy

Aromatherapy is the use of essential oils from plants or flowers as a therapy to improve physical and mental well-being. Aromatherapy can be used with other complementary treatments, such as massage or acupuncture, as well as general medical treatments. It can be a support with many ailments. In the case of cancer, it can help alleviate some symptoms or the effects of its treatment.

The most common way to use essential oils is inhalation or applying them to the skin in diluted form, but some can also be ingested. According to the National Cancer Institute, the only aromatherapy research with cancer patients has been to study the effects of essential oils on anxiety, nausea, vomiting and similar symptoms, and those results were positive. In my personal treatment, the aromas I used most were lavender, frankincense, lemongrass, lemon, orange and rosemary.

Reiki and Bioenergetic Balance

Reiki is an energy healing technique. There aren't many studies regarding its use in cancer treatment, but there are certainly indications that it can improve a person's mood and attitudes toward any disease. A study by oncology and psychology specialists from University of Huddersfield in England suggested that *reiki* can improve the quality of life of cancer patients by reducing their levels of anxiety, depression and fatigue. The benefits lasted up to two weeks after each session.[48]

There are various other modalities and therapies. I've simply shared the ones I used, along with nutritional supplements.

PREPARE YOUR GROUND

Here, in a summary way, are the measures I recommend and that may be useful if you want to begin a process of recovery, regardless of the illness.

- **Maintain an optimistic, positive attitude.** This doesn't mean that you're not in touch with your feelings or that you're not allowed to really experience them. Give your emotions space.
- **Share more with the people you most love.** The positive emotions generated by sharing also help you.
- **Vent your emotions and avoid holding them in.** Learn to express and process what happens to you.
- **Incorporate practices that promote tranquility and trust.** Uncontrolled emotions, especially fear, detach you from attunement to your healing ability so you lose balance and the coherent connection with your internal self. Fear triggers the alarms of the reptilian brain, generating the stress hormones, which counteract your ability to generate a proper recovery climate. When we're scared, our internal biological balance

changes, the immune system gets affected, defenses go down, and the prognosis gets worse. Without denying the reality of what's happening, don't sentence yourself. Work for the solution and trust.

- **Release your past and make peace with your history.** Drop all sense of blame or guilt. Get help if you need guidance. Reconcile yourself with what's happening to you, whatever you need to resolve. Forgive yourself and release the blame. Live with greater peace with yourself and others.

- **Practice retrospection.** Every night, take stock of what you've done. Bring your reactions and emotions to the conscious plane. Review what happened to you, how tired you got, how much you were present with yourself, etc. Through hindsight become aware of the rhythm of your life and propose to change habits so you can devote more time to your body, to give it the space you couldn't give it before and that may have led you to get sick.

- **Learn to manage stress.** Excessive stress leads into what's called sympathotonia, which inhibits the parasympathetic engagement which is needed for repair. A relaxed body and mind create a chemistry conducive to positive change of any kind.

- **Take rest time during the day.** Especially in the case of major illnesses, take at least 1-2 hours daily to rest in addition to the sleep hours at night. Focus on your healing and make this your priority. There can be nothing more important because life and its quality are at stake. Again, you must generate that state when the parasympathetic nervous system relaxes the body and inhibits many high functions, so more energy is available for the body to apply its healing resources. If your situation is one of prevention, then generally take at least half an hour in the middle of the day to rest and relax silently.

- **Respect and promote nighttime sleep.** Sleep not only allows you to rest, but also allows processes to be reversed and allows your body to repair. I suggest creating a suitable sleeping environment. Darken the room as much as you can. Sleep is essential for the improvement of any disease, especially diseases such as cancer, arthritis, fibromyalgia and kidney failure, among others.
- **Prioritize and begin what is absolutely necessary.** It's one thing to feel useless because you can't do everything you used to do and it's another thing to dedicate yourself to yourself. Taking care of you becomes your mission. You don't have to prove that you can do everything. Show yourself and your body how much you value it.
- **Read about light, funny subjects, watch humorous movies, or take in stories with good messages.** Avoid bloody, violent and stressful images.
- **Practice breathing exercises.** Restricted breathing may decrease your ability to heal.
- **Start the day by drinking water with lemon and maintain a good level of hydration by drinking natural water.** This practice helps eliminate toxins and facilitates the body's metabolic processes.
- **Check your diet; eat healthier and lighter.**
- **Avoid eating excessive quantities and, above all, monitor quality.** Favor raw foods: fruits and vegetables. Minimize or remove meats, depending on the condition. Remove sugar, refined flours, dairy and processed foods, because they increase inflammation. Check the utensils you cook with and avoid plastics and Teflon.
- **Chew well and take your time.** Rest a little after eating. Practice conscious feeding.
- **Avoid using microwaves.** Avoid electromagnetic contamination.

- **Detoxify yourself as much as you can.** Find out if, depending on your condition, you're a candidate for a full detox process assisted by a doctor. While you're finding out, start by eliminating most of the toxins within your reach. It starts with diet.
- **Consume detox foods:** ginger, lemon, apples, garlic, celery, linseed, pineapple, cucumber, parsley, nopal, aloe, fennel, turmeric, green tea, arugula and broccoli. All of these contain different components that help eliminate toxins.
- **Prepare purifying green juices, with a high chlorophyll content.** One of many combinations is: cucumber, celery, parsley, ginger and pineapple.
- **Take 2 tablespoons of olive oil on an empty stomach with 1 tablespoon of pure lemon juice.** It's an old folk remedy for the removal and expulsion of toxic residues from the liver.
- **Periodically apply enemas using purifying plants, oils, or organic coffee.** Coffee enemas help with liver detoxification, because of their choleretic action (increasing the volume of secretion of bile and solids from the liver).
- **Rinse your mouth with oil.** Sesame, sunflower seed or coconut oil is recommended, best if cold pressed. This is part of and accelerates a general detox process. It's an ancient ayurvedic practice from India written about by Dr. Karach.[49] If carried out two to three times daily, preferably before meals on an empty stomach, this can support the treatment of many diseases. Take a tablespoon of oil and rinse the mouth for 15–20 minutes. This practice is also known as oil pulling, *kavala* or *gundusha*.
- **Don't take medicines that aren't essential and prescribed.** Use mostly organic products, according to your options.

- **Maintain general hygiene and especially oral hygiene.** Check your teeth and dental repairs for any leaks, damaged teeth or fillings in poor condition in or bad positions. By having a healthy mouth, teeth, and gums you favor healing, and many interferences to healing can come from an unhealthy mouth. Floss your teeth. Keep a good toothbrush and use a tongue cleaner or a spoon.
- **Exercise regularly without exhausting yourself.** This practice maintains your cardiovascular health, improves your circulation, helps remove toxins and stimulates endorphins, relaxing your body.
- **Promote sweating.** The skin is the largest organ and is linked to detoxification. Vigorous exercise is one way to sweat. You can also do it by taking hot baths, steam baths or saunas for short periods. By exposing the pores to heat, they become enlarged and allow the impurities of the body to be released through the sebaceous glands. It also increases circulation and helps your body get rid of the excess fluid accumulated. Be careful to hydrate well when you do this.
- **Get massages and body therapies.** These improve your circulation and will help you eliminate waste and promote well-being.
- **Align yourself with nature.** The beach, the mountains, the great outdoors is excellent for fortifying and relaxation. If your physical conditions allow you to move freely, enjoy nature often. Enjoy it with small walks, get barefoot, breathe, go swimming. But beware of prolonged exposure to very strong sun in important periods of illness.
- **Disconnect from your mobile phone, social networks and constant exposure to the media.** Focus on yourself; now is your time. Avoid distracting yourself with what's not essential.

- **Practice inner silence and loving kindness to your-self.** Spend time alone, pamper yourself, do your best. You are the most important. Repeat healing expressions often, such as, "I take care of myself, I love myself, I give my best." Ask your body, "How can I please you today? How can I thank you and tell you that I care about you? How can I show you my own love?"

AND AFTER?

Even if you've finished your treatments, even if you're already in remission and your controls remain normal, continue with a plan. It's smart to keep doing everything that helps you to stay healthy. This keeps you on the anti-cancer path. If you've followed complementary treatments, consult your doctor and ask for a maintenance and supervision plan.

PART V

REVITALIZE

THOUSANDS OF YEARS AGO,
LONG BEFORE WESTERN
SCIENTISTS DISCOVERED
THE QUANTUM LAWS OF
THE UNIVERSE, THE ASIANS
ALREADY HONORED ENERGY
AS THE PRINCIPAL FACTOR
OF HEALTH AND WELL-BEING.

BRUCE LIPTON

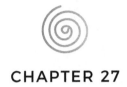

CHAPTER 27

REVITALIZE: LIGHT UP YOUR LIFE

Vitality and vital energy are the foundations of life. An evil cannot be cured when there is no life energy left in the body.

— HUANG TI

After having made a thorough *Review*, having *Removed* all kinds of toxins and initiated *Repair* on many levels, you're seeing evidence of positive changes. The fruits of these labors is a greater sense of vitality.

At the physical level your biology is energized. Your body's economy is becoming "profitable" because you're investing less extra effort in overloaded organs or systems. You save more energy and you generate more.

At the emotional level, you're handling things better. You can experience events with greater freedom, consciousness and a sense of ongoing connection. The awareness of your emotional intelligence with less drama and more responsible action is your welcome to the adult world. With this awareness, you can live more fully and with greater pleasure, creativity and positivity.

Your body is at the service of that which is essential to you, the spark of vital energy. Being vital, you can align yourself with your purposes and fulfill your life's mission, leaving behind the patterns and sabotages that used to pull you off your path and leave you feeling drained. Maybe you didn't even realize your lack of vitality until you recovered it and were back in the flow.

Inner strength, well-being and revitalization are activated by performing activities every day that allow for a stronger body-mind connection. You make significant changes and sustain them by turning those changes, practices and ways of seeing into your normal. Every day, your present becomes about following that routine of self-care and the quality it brings into a rhythm that flows naturally and joyfully. It springs from how you relate to yourself, to others and to your environment.

In essence, you tune in to life by making quality your norm. The changes you've made have become your way of life and not just a heroic contingency plan resorted to in the face of a crisis. This goes beyond what some colleagues have called "putting out fires." If we're only putting out fires, applying band-aids or crisis mode intervention, then it's very difficult to *Revitalize*. This is especially true in cases or conditions where there's already been deep damage. The proposal is clear: your habits make the difference. It's up to you to create the possibility of living longer with greater vitality, functional independence and enjoyment.

Revitalize is a consciousness where we naturally assume the practices of maintaining our state of energy. When you reach that state of consciousness and commitment, you can bring life to your years. If for some reason you disconnect from your personal care, you can resume those routines more quickly. There may be unexpected changes along the way, relapses, highs and lows as in the normal course of life. But you can deal with these things in a new way. If something unfortunate happens that's beyond your control, or some new learning, your body responds much better; you feel more resourceful in facing and figuring out what's going on. This, I can assure you, because when I found out I had cancer, I lived it. I realized I had a body that was well taken care of, so I had the resources which allowed me to respond from the vital force of my cells.

With greater connection to life you increase your confidence and belief that you can succeed and you see the signs that previously went unnoticed.

It's a conscious process of transforming old patterns. It's like you're recycling. Old patterns are recycled and their energy becomes the force to overcome obstacles and achieve goals. Sadness becomes a space to mourn but also to reflect and plan more sensibly. Fear translates into caring more and taking responsibility for your life. It embraces the opportunity to explore the unknown. Anger reinvents itself as a spirit of overcoming and meeting challenges. Pride becomes humility, compassion and empathy. Guilt becomes merit and recognition becomes conscience.

When you've regained the essential self, with a greater awareness of who you really are and your sense of purpose, your worth is established. You can experience life's polarities with the ability to stay focused on your path. You give your lights and shadows a healthy coexistence. You flow more with life and the movement it generates in you. It's a more present time and above all, more vital.

CHAPTER 28

YOU ARE ENERGY

"And life comes. It takes all its strength and momentum from the energetic seed of man and woman. Atoms become molecules; molecules become compounds; compounds translate into living matter; and suddenly the cell emerges, and splits into two, and into four and eight parts. And it multiplies in millions that at a miraculous moment begin to smile and breathe."

— SOPHIE HELLINGER

Energy is the essential life force that animates all life forms in the universe. The universe is a gigantic field of energy formed by the vibration of all that exists in within it. Human beings interact with this universal field through their own energy field, formed by different planes or energy frequencies.

Our body is made up of molecules and atoms, and what separates one atom from another is electromagnetic energy. Einstein, with his famous equation, $E=mc^2$, made a great contribution to the understanding of our energetic reality. Matter and energy are essentially interchangeable: energy gives rise to matter and matter gives rise to energy.

We also have the contributions of quantum physics, one of whose great movers was Max Planck, the Nobel Prize-winning physicist who also demonstrated that all matter originates and exists only by virtue of a force that vibrates the particles of an atom and holds them together. In other words, all reality is an energetic vibration.

In ancient Greece this energy was called *pneuma*, alluding to the wind or breath. In Polynesia it was *mana*. In the Old Testament, the Hebrews referred to it as the *ruah*, or "breath of life." The ancient Chinese called this energy *qi (chi)* and described it as invisible, silent and formless which permeates everything. The Chinese ideogram for *qi* depicts "the steam coming from the pot where the rice is being cooked."

This *qi* or vital energy manifests itself in the universe in different ways. It manifests itself in the sum total of all the energies of the cosmos, including gravity, magnetism, electricity, solar energy, radio waves and so forth. It also manifests as energy that nourishes all living organisms. For the living organism, *qi* is what electricity is for electrical equipment; without it, the equipment can't work. *qi* is what makes the difference between life and death.

Our bodies, as bodies of energy, need a certain vibration to stay vital and healthy. When that energy changes its vibratory level, it loses balance and causes a disruption of the flow in the body. As a result, this disruption becomes the basis of physical or psychological disorders. This can manifest initially at subtle levels, and usually imperceptibly. If it continues, it causes an energetic blockage that begins to affect the body-mind. This blockage prevents the proper circulation of energy and, though it may take years to materialize, can gradually lead to disease. It's important to keep this system as balanced as possible.

Balance is restored by activating one's vital energy. The life-force contains all the healing potential necessary to release blockages and recover the flow of energy. It can help restore health and physical and mental balance.

Energy medicines have a lot to contribute here. In the case of the TCM, one can recognize in a person's pulse, the color of their complexion or their tongue certain changes that alert you to an imbalance. Then you can begin to re-balance without having seen a symptom. This is the essence of preventive medicine.

Learning to perceive our energy is a way of getting to know ourselves better, reactivating our power and awakening and sharpening our senses. Moreover, when we begin to recognize our own energy, we recognize ourselves.

There are many ways to perceive and organize energy. At this point I resort to my knowledge of TCM as a way of showing connections and understanding the flow of energy. Also, it's one of the oldest documented energy models. It doesn't have scientific prestige in the West, but it has the endorsement of history. It has the endorsement of results and of its undeniable persistence through time as a resource. TCM was my gateway into the world of energy as a healing resource and it's been the mainstay of the work at Lunavital, the health center I founded over 26 years ago.

As a side note, in 1979, acupuncture was recognized by the WHO as an effective therapy for the treatment of at least 49 diseases and disorders, including anxiety and chronic stress. Thanks to more recent research, this list has been expanded.

Just as the physical body has blood vessels through which blood flows, there are channels in the energetic part of the body through which *qi* flows and is distributed. Energy moves through the body in the same way as electricity, following well-defined circuits. In TCM, these circuits are called channels or meridians. They form an invisible network that distributes *qi* to all of our tissues and organs.

There are 12 main channels – each associated with an important organ or vital function – as well as other secondary channels. When the circulation of energy ceases to be fluid, it stagnates and produces a situation where there's either a vacuum of energy or an overabundance. This imbalance of energy is the root of all our imbalances and the cause of disease. Moreover, in this tradition, the human being is an integrated energy system closely linked not only with other living systems, such as animals and plants, but also with the environment that surrounds it.

Through acupuncture, for example, TCM offers us an integrated approach that assesses the state of internal and external energies and makes symptoms understandable. The model presents us with the five mutable kingdoms or elements that correspond to the energy of water, wood, fire, earth and metal. These in turn correspond to certain organs or viscera, flavors, colors, foods, emotions and orientations. They form the basis for treating diseases with traditional energy concepts.

For instance, TCM correlates the connections between organs, tissues, emotions, orientation and climate with the concepts of the five elements, and so considers:

- Kidney and bladder energy can't be separated from bones, cold, fear, winter, hearing and the salty.
- The liver and gallbladder are related to spring, wind, sight, anger, muscles and the acidic.
- The heart and small intestine are related to summer, heat, sadness and joy, the circulatory system and the bitter.
- The spleen and stomach are related to transitions between the seasons, humidity, reflection and obsession and the sweet.
- The lung and large intestine are linked with the fall, drought, sadness, the skin, the sense of smell and the spicy.

Obviously, TCM views the organs and emotions as intimately connected. Organs may also be affected by diet, changes in one's environment or habits or hereditary factors.

Through energy medicine, a modern disorder like anxiety is seen as an imbalance in the functioning of different organs. Accordingly, worry and excessive mental work are associated with disturbances at the energy level of the spleen/stomach and the earth. A lack of vitality and enthusiasm, restlessness, depression, insomnia and despair are symptoms of a heart/small intestine energy disorder. Some emotional symptoms, such as anger, indecision, resentment, frustration, irritability and bitterness are related to the liver/gallbladder. Pain, melancholy, longing, sadness and attachment are linked to the large lung/intestine. Fear, anxiety, an extreme sense of responsibility, rigid self-demand, insecurity and isolation are all related to an imbalance in the kidneys/bladder.

What I'm emphasizing here is how the energetic body and the dense or physical body affect each other. When we heal one, the other also heals.

Dr. Wilhelm Reich spoke of this same energy, which he called *orgonic*. His revolutionary and controversial energy research was a profound influence on all the Bioenergy schools, as they deal with psychological conflicts from or with the body. In bioenergetics, our pre-existing emotions, conflicts we've experienced and losses we've suffered – in other words, all of our previous affective relationships – determine what we are today. Once again, the story is imprinted on our body. But it can be released through the muscular, energetic or breathing exercises of the bioenergetic approach.[50]

Simply stated, energy is force in motion and action. As to biological energy, this is the force in action capable of producing both emotions and physiological events.

This brings us back to quantum physics and its concept of energy leads us at the atomic and subatomic levels. Thanks to quantum physics it's been verified scientifically that anything we're able to perceive with our senses, be it solid, liquid or gas, in its most infinitesimal parts, is made up of groups of particles that in turn are made up of smaller particles called *quanta*. A quantum is the smallest particle a physical entity can possess; a single packet of matter or energy. So as physical beings we are energy. Everything is pure energy. And these tiny units of energy, the quanta, can exist both as waves and particles and flow from one form to the other. The only time they manifest as particles is when we're looking at them.

I've brought this up because it leads to another dimension of energy work. Much has been said about the power of intention or the power of the mind and heart in healing work. It's nothing new. But let's enliven that in a personal, practical way with the "quantum perspective" by saying, "What we are depends on how we perceive ourselves." In other words, if we can change our perception, we can transform our energy and so transform what we are.

The foundation of this approach is work with our quanta, our units of energy which can pass from the invisible to the visible and vice versa and which can become a biological cell, a thought, a feeling or a part of our soul. This is our connection to a unity of body, mind and spirit. It allows us to open ourselves to the transformative power of our totality.

Many have said that we are spiritual beings passing through a material experience. We are matter and spirit at the same time. These two aspects of being are powerfully interrelated and can therefore affect each other in a positive or negative way. It's in our hands to manage how each is affected.

ACTIONS FOR A R.E.A.L. LIFE

Sensing *qi* in your hands. *Qi* can be activated. It can be concentrated, generated and moved at will and you can do it as auto-therapy. It can also help you feel more connected. Start breathing and releasing tensions. Breathing is your support right now. Keep it flowing, breathing as fully as possible without forcing it. Let your arms relax and hang at the sides of your body. Take three full breaths and concentrate on your hands, on the center of your palms. Inhale gently and, without losing focus on the palms of your hands, slowly raise your hands to the height of your chest. Now turn your palms down and exhale slowly as you gradually lower your hands. Stay focused on your breathing. When your arms are hanging again at your side, breathe normally and try to feel the sensation the exercise has produced. The sensation of the energy flow of manifests with heat, tingling or a slight vibration. It's just a matter of bringing it to consciousness. Repeat this twice more.

Stimulating the energy (*ting* points). Massage your fingers to stimulate your body and all the energy. Start by stimulating the distal part of your fingers and toes, especially at the nail angles of each finger and each toe. Stay aware of your breathing. With this you activate the channels of energy both from where it springs and where it changes in polarity. Then give a massage to the whole of each finger of one hand, then the other and then the toes of each foot. Keep breathing fully, softly and consciously . . .

Expanding your energy. First close your eyes, breathe and feel the body's energy. Take a mental tour of your body, breathing and slowly relaxing each part. Now smile. Smile internally and begin to touch your body, passing your hands gently over it while still smiling. Go to whatever part of your body feels most in need and gently rest your hands there, relaxed. Smile internally and generate that healing energy for your body, for your cells and for that part of you that needs more right now. Breathe, imagining the light and bring it to that place there while you smile at it. Stay there as long as you feel like it.

CHAPTER 29

CONCERNING STRESS

"Stress is being here wanting to be there."
— ECKHART TOLLE

Who doesn't have stress these days?

Stress was the topic of my first public workshops and my first experiences as a facilitator back in 1995. I've studied stress for many years and from various points of view and it's something I'm passionate about. I've gradually incorporated many new experiences to my understanding of the topic, some of which were personal and some I encountered through my work with patients.

Stress has been called "the disease of modernity" or, as per the title of Daniel López Rosetti's book, *Stress, The Epidemic of the XXI Century*.[51] Modern life, with everything it offers, tends to bring frequent stress to our lives, even in childhood. Still it's not very easy to define. For many, even in the medical profession, stress is still a myth.

Walter Cannon was a neurologist and researcher whose studies proceeded from the hypothesis that to be healthy, human beings must maintain an internal balance, a homeostasis (which is our normal range of elementary physiological function). But in case of intense change or stimuli, a process of rearrangement occurs through the endocrine and the autonomic nervous system. This is stress, says Cannon, and it can be generated by charged events and situations, either physical or psychological in nature.[52]

Hans Selye departed from Cannon's advances and discovered that his patients had certain biological constants regardless of the type of stress or illness they suffered. From this observation, he developed a definition of stress based not on the stimulation but on the particular individual's response during stressful situations. So Selye contributed the notion of a precondition which determines how each individual incorporates, processes and responds to stress.[53]

There are situations that are in themselves generally stressful. There's even a stress classification list that's used as a reference. However, the response to that general stress will depend on the person's history, what they've recorded as trauma, their impacting events and predispositions, as well as their coping mechanisms and current experiences. Other influences will include the person's records of positive emotions, their emotional base and physical fortitude.

In simple terms, as outlined by Selye, stress has to do with both internal and external "overloads" and our responsiveness to them. Hence, the same burden can be borne differently by different people.[54]

In addition, comparative studies of responses to situations that are considered universally stressful found that not all people are stressed in the same way. For some an event can be stressful; for others not. Again, this depends on various factors, such as the person's perspective on life, their levels of self-demand and demands of others, their expectations, their emotional platform, adaptability and so on. But there's always a point for every individual where things are so charged that eventually, whether emotionally, mentally or corporally, stress manifests itself in some way.

I'd like to point out that a little stress that keeps us on our toes is positive. It helps us pay attention and stimulates our reflexes so we can respond quickly to a threat or be ready to face a challenge. It even gives us motivation. In these cases, once the stress trigger situation has passed, the nervous system quickly returns to its baseline.

But stress is not always a reaction to immediate or current events. Long-term situations can produce sustained stress that, regardless of the intensity, ends up causing changes in the nervous system, the hormonal system and the immune system. It can even deplete the body's reserves. This happens almost imperceptibly, as most people adapt before any noticeable changes occur. We have a design that naturally protects us from change, because our physiology continually returns us to balance. Eventually, however, the body can lose the ability to respond, causing a collapse and the appearance of imbalance, symptoms or disease. This has been studied extensively by psychoneuroimmunology, which examines the interaction between psychological processes and the nervous and immune systems.

In a state of calm, the frontal cortex of the brain is activated. Interestingly, this is the part where creativity and the ability to make fresh, new decisions reside. In a state of stress, brain circulation leaves the front and concentrates on the back of the brain, where survival mechanisms learned in the past are activated. In the back of the brain is where we keep the memory and files of past experiences, including our ancestral and primitive past. Our stressful lifestyle keeps us in the back of our brains most of the time, leaving the front part vacant. So, with our reptilian brain activated, it's as if we're in a constant struggle for survival. Regardless of their intensity, we mostly face these long-term pressures with no help, because they're "normal." However, they keep our brains functioning in a primitive way.

Here's a list of typical stresses:

- Being always in a hurry and on the move, with no time to rest or relax.
- Being the victim of intimidation or exposed to violence or physical injury.
- Tense relationships, family conflicts, a relationship break-up, the death of a loved one.
- Work situations: a lack of work, conflicts at work, having lots of employees.
- Excessive responsibilities.
- Lack of proper rest.
- An unhealthy diet.

Some stresses are extreme and for those you need attention; you should seek professional help. For instance, PTSD (post-traumatic stress disorder) is a strong reaction that can occur in people who've gone through an extreme trauma like a serious car accident, a natural disaster, a rape or assault, the sudden death of a close relative and so on.

There are also people with deep anxiety problems who are extremely reactive to normal stress, turning small difficulties into larger crises. Overcoming anxiety disorders usually requires professional attention.

STRESS TO THE VITAL ORGANS

I want to mention this type of stress, because we mention it a lot in consultations when we explain to a patient what happens to their internal organs. As I've said, stressful factors can be psychological or physical. Both can end up causing pathological changes at the physical level and causing stress at the organ level.

From a physiological point of view, the organism always tends to balance. No matter what's going on inside of it or outside, there are variables that must always remain constant and the body needs them balanced to function optimally. To achieve this, the organism resorts to dynamic mechanisms that help it to return to normalcy, or homeo-stasis. This also applies to what happens outside and inside our cells.

When a body has been under stress for a long time, the system of self-regulation gets weaker and it becomes increasingly difficult for it to maintain balance. I compare it to a company with a department that's consistently unprofitable. Due to that one department's deficit, the company has to make an ever greater effort to balance the budget. If the deficit isn't compensated, the higher cost of maintaining that department can put the whole company at risk. So it is with the body. Sometimes the cost of keeping it running is high, but we don't realize the stress it puts on our organs to keep in balance. In these cases, which are increasingly frequent in modern life, our "biological budget" is in the red.

Chronic stress, then, is one of the environmental factors associated with the emergence of various pathologies: cardiovascular disorder, hypertension and depression of the immune system. Chronic stress also affects neural functioning and can have serious consequences, such as increased risk of suicide or emotional disorders.

No matter what causes our stress, if we also contribute to the problem with unhealthy physical behaviors, the bodily stress worsens. Examples of these behaviors are eating food loaded with toxic ingredients, being sedentary, not resting well, breathing contaminated air, staying in difficult postures long-term, exposure to excessive noise, overexertion beyond one's physical limits and the like. All of these, in addition to being stressful for the body, lower our overall energy level, which weakens our ability to respond.

STRESS IN CHILDREN

Many still consider it a myth, but the reality is that children also get stressed out. It's common these days to find overstressed children – especially in urban areas – because they're usually overburdened with activities, pressured to be competitive and simultaneously caught up in their parents' stressful lifestyle. The causes are many, but aside from the topics of diet, sleep patterns or dysfunctions in the family dynamic, I'd like simply to draw attention to the issue in families, schools and communities.

These are among the most common causes of stresses in children:

- Numerous extracurricular activities with little play and leisure time.
- Excessive amounts of homework.
- Ongoing situations at school caused by learning problems.
- Fears, phobias, insecurities.
- Issues of conflict, disagreements or unclear rules between parents.
- Physical or psychological burdens corresponding to adults.
- Abuse, bullying or harassment of any nature.

Many studies already support the notion that stresses are transmitted from parents to children, not only via their environment, but also through inheritance. Obviously, mothers and fathers have tremendous influence on their children. Eric Nestler of the Mount Sinai School of Medicine in New York, suggests the high possibility that if their parents are exposed to significant stress, children are at increased risk for stress-related disorders.[55]

THE CLASSIC PHASES OF STRESS

One of Hans Selye's great contributions is his famous theory, the general adaptation syndrome, in which he outlines three stages of stress.[56] I find it useful to share and comment on:

The Alarm Phase

This is the phase we see most. It occurs in every person when the body perceives and begins to defend itself against a stressful, threatening agent. At this stage the body initially responds without us even realizing it, and it can present various symptoms.

In our first, rapid reaction, the respiratory rate increases, some muscles contract and the pulse accelerates. After the stressful situation passes, everything returns to normal. This can happen not only in the face of extraordinary events, such as hearing bad news, an accident or a heated discussion. It can also happen in everyday life when we have emotional conflicts, work overload, a tense work environment, in traffic, with time-pressure, multi-tasking, noise, self-imposed pressures, limits on communication, etc.

Even when the body lets go of these routine stresses and relaxes again, it has still been submitted to the effects of a minor crisis. With regular repetition, these effects eventually carry risks, even worse than those caused by a singular or occasional more significant event.

The Resistance Phase

In this phase, there's so much repetition of the stressful agent that the body ends up adapting and the symptoms disappear. I compare it to the constant, uniform noise produced by some electrical equipment that's kept running all the time. It's called white noise and we adapt to it so successfully that soon we don't notice it anymore, unless it suddenly stops. Then to our surprise we feel relieved. This happens in the body with all kinds of stressful elements.

Many people who come for a consultation say they don't have any stress because they don't feel it. Actually, in most of these cases they've adapted to the routine overload and don't realize it. When they list everything they do each day and all that's happened to them, and even more so when we begin to examine the body, we see the consequences. The body pays a high price to adapt and stay in balance with a permanent overload.

The phase of resistance is responsible for organic stress. It's the internal organs that "go the extra mile" to allow us to keep functioning and maintain the internal balance. It's as if we have a truck with a capacity to carry 20 tons and we load it with 30 tons. It can manage 30 tons, but it wears out faster than it would with normal use. Sooner or later, it just breaks down.

The sad thing is that most people are completely unaware of this and think they're fine. They live so automatically that they don't think to question themselves. When a symptom appears - a pain, a heart attack or an illness - they don't connect it to their stress because they weren't even aware of it. It's often been my experience in consultations that when people are highly skeptical when stress is indicated as the possible cause of their condition. They don't believe it's possible.

The side effects of this kind of stress impact the energy system and vital organs so slowly that they're virtually imperceptible. So for a long time the person feels normal. The autonomous nervous system and all the automatic compensation systems work on their own to maintain balance as much as possible. Eventually, some symptoms begin to appear, but most people also adapt to them, until they get worse.

Here are some of these symptoms:

· Tiredness (easier than before). This is followed by a fatigue that doesn't go away with rest.
· Occasional headaches that return more and more often.
· Circulatory problems, heaviness in the legs, maybe varicose veins.

- Digestive problems: abdominal distension, slow digestion, constipation, stomach pains.
- Insomnia, sleep disturbance, difficulty resting.
- Lack of concentration, lack of focus.
- Muscle contractures in the neck, back and lumbar area, which do not relax with rest.
- Distraction, occasional memory failure.
- Pessimism, a feeling of failure.

The Exhaustion Phase

If a significant stress continues for a long time, there comes a point when the body can't continue the effort to adapt and the energies run out. There's a break in the internal balance and the recovery processes. Then the immune system is affected and disease appears. If the damage is very significant, the life may even be at risk. If it's less serious, the process may be partially reversible, though perhaps with ongoing consequences. Some examples of these include high blood pressure, heart attack, stroke, ulcer, cancer and infections.

In short, the body's response to acute stress is more protective and adaptive, while the response to chronic stress produces a biochemical imbalance resulting in immunosuppressive alterations. The alterations lead to the development of inflammatory diseases, fatigue caused by the exhaustion of the adrenal glands, metabolic imbalances including obesity, type 2 diabetes and cardiovascular diseases.

There's plenty of scientific evidence of the negative impact of chronic stress on the nervous system, the endocrine system and the immune system and its role in causing a large number of diseases. Given all of the above, any discussion of stress management has to include a serious consideration of lifestyle. And this should bring us to ask ourselves, "What is quality of life?" It should push us to revise our reductive perspective.

Therefore, in addition to the usual factors that make up a healthy lifestyle, we should include fostering emotional intelligence and the development of coping mechanisms. Some examples of these are: relaxation programs, body consciousness, meditation, mindfulness, visualization and breathing. Of course, these things can only be added if one's daily activities are adjusted to make time. This means we may have to prioritize and reorganize our agenda.

MORE COHERENCE, LESS STRESS

This brings us back to the notion of personal coherence. I'll try to explain it in a simple way through the Chinese ideogram Wang, which means emperor. I still use this ideogram as a way of personal review. In ancient times, the emperor was the "son of heaven" and seen as a kind of heir and representative of heaven on earth. His words were orders and considered sacred decrees, because he was viewed as a superior being.

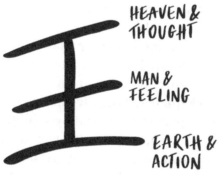

The ideogram representing the emperor consists of three horizontal lines or strokes and one vertical stroke. The three horizontal strokes correspond as follows:

- **Upper stroke:** Sky. The emperor is in contact with Heaven. It represents his thoughts, which are heavenly inspired.

- **Middle stroke:** Humanity. The emperor is also human and therefore feels and has emotions. So this represents feelings and relationships with others.
- **Lower stroke:** Earth. The emperor dwells on earth. This represents his actions and concrete things, the material world, the body.
- **Vertical stroke:** Connects all three worlds, expressing a balance between them. The emperor communicates and integrates the three by uniting the spiritual and intangible world of heaven with the manifested, concrete world of earth.

The emperor is in coherence. His thoughts are in tune with heaven, which he communicates and connects with related feelings and turns into consistent action. There's harmony between what he thinks, feels and does and all three levels move in the same direction. Thus he thinks, feels and acts without any conflicts that threaten his truth. Therein lies his perfection and his health. He's the archetype of balance on all three levels.

For me, this ideogram is an invitation to review my own coherence. Likewise, I invite you to review yours, so you can take the proper steps to manage your stress and live a life with more quality. Truly, whatever you do, whatever you include as part of your healing will go beyond being just a strategy or a burden forcing you to take up a bunch of practices. It will become the manifestation of coherence in your life. That's why these practices are called steps of coherence.

Speaking of coherence, I can't leave out cardiac coherence. This is a recent term, which we owe to studies developed by the HeartMath Institute in California. To summarize, this is a group of scientists who've demonstrated that emotions impact the heart rate. And they've named that effect the CPV or cardiac pulse variability.[57]

CPV analysis is a tool to measure nervous system dynamics, which are also a key indicator of stress levels. If a person is referred to as having high cardiac coherence it means that their CPV is balanced. It indicates an efficient state of psychological functioning in which the nervous, cardiovascular, endocrine and immune systems are working harmoniously and well. It's the basis of optimal performance and health.

The time between our heartbeats varies subtly beat to beat. When there's stress that variation is greater and more irregular. Based on this knowledge, the idea is to train one's heart to beat more regularly, thus reducing stress levels and their consequences. This notion proceeds from the fact that the heart has its own neural circuit interconnected with the emotional brain, which controls the emotions and the body's physiology. This circuit consists of tens of thousands of neurons that act as "miniature brains," each capable of having their own perceptions, modifying their responses accordingly and even transforming themselves as a result of their experiences.

Not only does the heart have this semi-autonomous system of neurons, it's also a small hormone factory. It harbors its own adrenaline reserve to use when it needs to perform at its maximum capacity. It also secretes and regulates the release of ANF, a hormone that regulates blood pressure. And it has its own reserve of oxytocin, the hormone responsible for bonding, compassion, kindness and love. All of these hormones act directly on the brain and greatly influence our organism.

When we're in "stress mode," our body isn't synchronized because our emotions are imbalanced. This causes a disorder in the heart rate and nervous system that blocks or inhibits the cerebral cortex or rational brain.

Emotions such as anger, anxiety, sadness and even banal worries provoke irregularity in the heart rate and cause disorder.

In contrast, positive emotions create harmony in the nervous system and heart rhythm, facilitating fluidity at the cerebral level while the rest of the body's systems are synchronized in the state that's been called coherence. Emotions such as joy, gratitude and, above all, love are conducive to coherence.

Coherence gives us mental clarity and the ability to make better decisions, so it makes it easier for us to deal with any stressful situation. By learning to control our heart, we regulate our emotional brain and vice versa. The strongest relationship between the heart and the emotional brain is established through the autonomous peripheral nervous system; that is, the part of the nervous system that regulates the functioning of all our organs.

To enter the path of coherence, first you must be able to recognize what's happened to you and what you need. If you've done that, congratulations, you've taken the first step. The second step is not to judge yourself. If you start an internal dialogue of complaints about what you have and haven't done, self-criticisms and self-blame, you'll only drain more energy and generate more stress. Remember, at each step we can act from whatever level of awareness we have. The time is now to start your plan of action, your commitment to yourself to live in better health.

The art of managing stress is the art of living well. It's perfected through practice, as you incorporate behaviors that become organic habits in your daily life instead of things you only resort to under pressure. Maintaining anti-stress practices, even when you feel calm, will help you to handle the difficult times that may arise.

ACTIONS FOR A R.E.A.L. LIFE

Avoid overloading yourself. If you feel stressed out, prioritize and eliminate some activities.
Learn to say both yes and no. Set healthy boundaries by taking care of yourself. Also learn to ask for help or support from others. Develop the art of delegating.

Learn to relax. You can find helpful guided relaxation exercises online. Take time to enjoy activities that calm you and make you happy. Watch a good movie, read a book, enjoy a hobby, play with your kids or a pet (if you have them) or take a relaxing bath.

Improve your cardiac coherence. Start with slow, deep breaths. Focus on rhythmic, complete breaths until it's easy and natural. Focus on your heart and chest and imagine breathing through the heart. Continue slowly, deeply and just be aware of the air moving in and out and visualize your heart. Continue for as long as it takes to feel at ease.

Defend your rest hours. Improve your sleep quality. Aromatherapy might help.

Increase your resilience. That's the ability to recover from traumatic or difficult situations. Also, learn to see challenges as opportunities. It's easier if you cultivate good sense of humor.

Live in the present. Try not to anticipate and worry.

Identify your personality. Some personalities tend to emphasize perfectionism, self-demands and anxiety. You can become addicted to burdens and living in tension.

Exercise regularly and in moderation.

CHAPTER 30

MORE EXERCISE, MORE HEALTH!

"Our nature is in motion. Absolute rest is death".
— BLAISE PASCAL

At a young age I was never an athlete. I used to do some intermittent exercise as a young adult but never with real commitment until just before I turned 40. Then I entered a very stressful period in my life and started walking and jogging every day in the early morning. With discipline and persistence, jogging led to running, which eventually led me to become a marathoner. These days, I run to stay healthy and I combine running with yoga because I really enjoy it. For me, these two activities are complementary and sacred.

You've no doubt heard from various sources that movement is health. It's well established that exercise is essential for a life of the highest quality and if you exercise regularly you definitely generate significant benefits that will allow you to enjoy a longer, healthier life. But recent studies into both epigenetics and the elongation of telomeres have confirmed this in new ways. Simply put, among the various actions you have at hand to prevent illness, boost energy, reverse chronic conditions and impact your overall well-being, physical exercise has an important role.

Since ancient times, physical activity has been associated with people's health. Throughout history the longevity of certain populations has been related to adequate nutrition and active lifestyles. It's been clearly demonstrated that properly performed physical exercise promotes health in numerous clinical and epidemiological studies.

It should also be noted that physical exercise is important not only to restore health, but to preserve it. This is why exercise is officially recommended for healthy people as well as for patients of various diseases. In many such cases, physical exercise complements traditional treatments for patients of any age and even reduces mortality. Regardless of your condition, exercise is also for you.

Regular physical exercise is an established recommendation for the prevention and treatment of the chief modifiable cardiovascular risk factors. These include diabetes mellitus, hypertension and dyslipidemia (high blood fats). Performing physical activity of moderate intensity for a minimum of 30 minutes five days per week or of high intensity for a minimum of 20 minutes three days per week, improves functional capacity and is associated with reductions in incidence of cardiovascular disease. If you decide on a more intense exercise routine with greater cardiovascular impact, I always suggest you get a cardiac check-up as a precaution.

Physical exercise naturally stimulates many mechanisms that protect the individual against premature aging and decrepitude. For the elderly, it definitely and effectively contributes to their quality of life and relative independence. Regular, continuous physical exercise for elderly people with chronic diseases and associated disabilities has produced significant results. In many cases, by the tenth week, muscle strength is doubled, walking speed, strength and balance are improved and bone density is increased.

If this can be achieved in the elderly, whose capacity for cellular response is diminished, often with deterioration, it should be obvious that in younger people, more forceful and faster change is even more possible. This means that no matter how old you are, exercise is also for you.

Now, let me warn against excessive exercise or over-training. Each body is different but overtraining is the result of exercise that is extreme for a given individual's physiological condition and usual training habits combined with insufficient time for the body to rest and recover. Remember, the body needs to move, yet it also needs rest, nutrition and sleep. Overtraining causes oxidative stress, damage to muscle cells and the cells responsible for their repair, which slows down recovery. For an extreme athlete, professional supervision is always recommended. The best thing is to start slowly, following a program of gradual increase until you get in shape.

Here's a summary of the consensus of health benefits from exercise:

- Reduces your risk of developing common vascular and metabolic disorders such as coronary heart disease, heart attack, hypertension, non-insulin dependent diabetes.
- Prevents you from being overweight and obese and also helps overcome numerous health issues.
- Strengthens your structures: bones, cartilage, ligaments, tendons and improves the function of your skeletal muscle system.
- Reduces gastric symptoms such as constipation and the risk of colon cancer.
- Increases your lung capacity.
- Promotes overall physical performance, giving you greater energy and vitality.
- Improve reflexes and motor coordination.

- On a psychological level, it has calming and antidepressant effects, it brings a feeling of well-being and lowers stress.
- Prevents insomnia and regulates sleep.
- Lengthens your telomeres and therefore your quality of health and your life.

These are some of the benefits. And though I'm sharing medical information and research results, as far as I'm concerned the most important thing is that you get excited about taking the first step and commit yourself to a regular exercise discipline, appropriate for your condition. You may say, "I don't have time," "I don't have energy," or "I'm too stressed right now to start." But let me tell you, this is the moment to start: when you least want to or feel overwhelmed. Exercising will change your life, decrease your reactivity to stress and even improve your mood.

You know the benefits of exercise. It's time now to start and make it a part of your life. I encourage you to find a physical activity that you enjoy and can get excited about. Find something that's not an imposition but rather something you do with pleasure.

ACTIONS FOR A R.E.A.L. LIFE

Identify what you like to do as an exercise and whether you prefer open or closed spaces.

Check what's better for your current condition. You can check it with your health guide.

Identify a way to start that's easier and faster for you, so it's harder to make excuses.

Find a location that's close to you and isn't hard to get to.

Find a group so you can do your exercise with company and support.

Make sure you have the right kind of shoes and basic exercise clothes. As you proceed, you'll figure out better what works for you.

Dance, walk, jog, swim, ride a bike, whatever you like best. Do it and enjoy it.

CHAPTER 31

BREATHE LIFE

"Air is your food and your medicine."

— ARISTOTLE

Breathing is a process common to all life forms, since the chemical basis of life essentially consists of an oxidation of tissues. Our arrival into this life is marked by our first inhalation and the end is marked with an exhalation. It's a natural function. But I include it here as a health practice because for millennia it's been a tool to support well-being and quality of life.

The influence of breathing on emotional states is well known. Likewise, our emotions impact our respiration. Everything is reflected in the breath. Joy makes you breathe deeply and dilates the chest. Sadness bows the head and the back by exerting a braking action on the sympathetic system so the heart is insufficiently oxygenated. Hence the phrase, "it weighs on the heart."

For thousands of years, various traditions maintained that our respiration is the only vital function we can voluntarily influence. They considered the nutrition we absorb through breathing equal in importance to food. They also understood that just as our emotional states alter our breathing, we can positively affect our moods and our body through conscious, directed breathing.

In principle, breathing is a matter of science, but in practice it's an art. It's essential to learn to breathe optimally and to do so daily to strengthen our organic capabilities. It's also essential for learning how to control ourselves and regain our calm in stressful situations.

In addition to increasing our vitality, with optimal breathing we can also activate blood, lymphatic and nervous circulation. This is not only because of the nutritional contribution of the air we inhale, but also because breathing helps eliminate toxins and wastes from our body.

Breathing is also important for increasing physical endurance and the ability to relax the body or center ourselves. Clearly, breathing helps give us a better quality of life and general well-being.

Basically, there are two types of functional breathing: the cleanser and the energizer. The cleansing breath focuses more on the exhalation and detoxifies the body. The energizer concentrates more on inhalation; it collects and accumulates vital energy. For each of these basic functions there are numerous variants with different specific effects.

Although most people usually don't pay much attention to the way they breathe, everyone spontaneously practices both kinds of breathing throughout the day, whenever the toxins in the blood reach a critical level or the energy begins to wane. An example of a spontaneous cleansing breath is the sigh: a rapid inhale followed by a forced, long exhale. The yawn is an example of spontaneous energetic breathing: a long, slow deep inhale, which is briefly retained in the lungs and then expelled with a relatively brief exhale.

Breathing, can also be shallow or deep. What distinguishes normal shallow respiration from deep abdominal respiration is the function of the diaphragm. The diaphragm is a strong flexible muscle membrane that separates the chest cavity from the abdominal cavity. When the lungs expand, they push the diaphragm down. When they contract, they pull the diaphragm into the chest cavity. In this way, the diaphragm plays a crucial role in the respiratory process.

What predominates among adults today is shallow pectoral or chest breathing, thanks to ignorance, sedentary life-styles, indiscriminate use of tobacco, environmental pollution, constipation and other factors. This breathing basically only fills the middle and upper section of the lungs, using the intercostal muscles to widen the upper part of the rib cage, which decreases the air pressure in the lungs and the outside air enters by suction. Breathing like this, the lower, largest section of the lungs isn't fully used.

Clavicular respiration is even less efficient. In this type of breathing, the clavicles are simply raised to open the narrow upper section of the lungs and the middle and lower sections of the lungs are barely used. The breaths must be rapid to compensate for the deficit of air. This kind of breathing is common with states of high anxiety or tension and also with women in advanced gestation, due to the compression exerted by the gravid uterus on the diaphragm. It's also characteristic of asthmatics and those with emphysema.

Full abdominal or diaphragmatic breathing uses all three sections of the lungs in a smooth and continuous expansion from the bottom up. First, the air is breathed into the lower section, allowing the diaphragm to dilate into the abdominal cavity. Then the intercostal muscles go into action to open the rib cage and fill the middle of the lungs with air. The inhalation ends with a small final effort that slightly lifts the clavicles to bring air to the narrow upper section of the lungs.

Diaphragmatic breathing significantly increases respiratory performance by reducing by more than half the number of inhalations and exhalations per minute. It conserves vital energy, works the heart less and causes a significant increase in blood circulation, bringing more oxygen to the whole body.

Under normal conditions, we perform 12 to 16 breaths per minute, though this frequency decreases during sleep and increases with physical exertion. That's the normal range. It's important to remember, however, when we begin to direct our own breathing that each body has its own rhythm.

ACTIONS FOR A R.E.A.L. LIFE

It's important to perform each phase correctly and to link them gently. In addition to protecting us from other particles, the tissues lining the nasal cavity and sinuses specialize in capturing the energy of the air. They also moisten the incoming air and adjust its temperature. So in these breathing exercises inhalation should be through the nose.

Breathing in 4 tempos.
The exercise consists of 4 fundamental phases for which 4 positions can be taken: standing, sitting, lying, walking.

Inhale.
Hold the breath.
Exhale.
Pause.

Inhale four times on a count of 4.
Hold the breath for a count of 4.
Exhale on a count of 6.
Pause for a count of 2.

Short breathing exercise to improve vitality: Take 4 short, audible breaths and 1 long breath. Repeat 4 times to reach a count of 20. Do this in the morning especially, but no more than twice per day.

PART VI

RESIGNIFY

HOW SMALL MY HANDS
ARE . . . IN RELATION TO
EVERYTHING THAT LIFE
HAS GIVEN ME.

RAMÓN J. SENDER

CHAPTER 32

RESIGNIFY: DISCOVER NEW COLORS

"Your life is your story. Write it well. Edit it often. "
— SUSAN STATTAM

Signification is the process of giving something a name or meaning. It's also the result of that process: the name or the meaning itself. To *Resignify* then, is to give something new meaning or significance or a new name. In the context of my approach, to *Resignify* is to find the positive in something difficult or painful you've experienced or are going through. It's finding the brilliance of the diamond in the rough.

Every new conflict or crisis in our lives is an opportunity and an invitation to really look at something, and that something is screaming to be looked at. It's the gift of a new starting point to continue our interior work and turn the event into a source of transformation.

There's a well-worn phrase that for me remains valid and applicable: "It's not what happens to you, it's what you do with what happens to you." You can be inspired by others; they can make you think or provoke an emotional response. But when you open your heart to what happens to you, it's something you conquer within yourself. From there you can change your attitude and really examine it. You can find connections, synchronicities and answers and everything begins to make new sense. When physical problems arise you meet your biological needs. You do what you need to do for your body, either by following the advice of your health care provider or applying your own knowledge if it's something you can handle on your own. At the same time, through the steps I've proposed, you can learn to look for what might be behind the problem or event. You can learn to read the message and focus on real healing, which occurs when you access all of your levels, including the dimensions of the soul.

This new phase allows you to make proactive decisions for your greatest good. You can do this from a place of serenity, sustained by the strength of having overcome something within you. You feel that you fully own your own process and sense the opportunities now within reach. You've entered the space of inner renewal and all of your energy is accessible. Yet you proceed with humility and a sense of human vulnerability. From now on, nothing will be the same. From this foundation, you have the opportunity to rewrite your story.

The idea is to give space in your heart to any situation you have to face, be it physical or emotional, in your relationships or work or in any of your roles. Regardless of how complex the situation might be and whatever pain it may bring, you can come to see it with love and respect. This is because you know that you fulfill a greater purpose and that knowing allows you to move forward with awareness, acceptance and dignity.

I lived all of this in a powerful way with cancer.It was the toughest lesson I faced, the most difficult thing to *Resignify*. But as I accomplished that, it exponentially reinforced my sense of intimate contact with myself, my body and my essence. I interact differently now with my body. I value it in its true sense as a temple so I take care of it with re-newed consciousness. Behind the cancer, behind the sense of threat and the suspense of uncertainty, I was able to find the blessing. I was able to open myself to a state in which two words kept resonating and I repeated them a thousand times: "Yes" and "Thank you!"

I assure you that when you *Resignify*, you come to see life differently. Life becomes an ongoing encounter of new roads that allow you a richer and deeper journey. You re-value life by recognizing who you are, your roots, your his-tory and your individual being with its lights and shadows. You value it, you accept it as it is and from there you value and accept everything else.

It's a state of consciousness in which the internal ob-server is active and alert; the intuition and a sense of connection with everything are present. A way of under-standing and processing what happens comes to you and nothing is alien. Everything belongs to you and you are 100% responsible for all that happens to you. You learn to look at the opportunities, the good fortune and lessons that every experience brings you and you become the protago-nist of your story. You allow yourself to see that something else, that wake-up call that appears in the form of pain, suf-fering or illness. You go through the pain, feel it, live it and let it pass through you. You don't try to get rid of it or evade it by anesthetizing yourself. You live it with your whole be-ing, feeling a sense of higher assistance. You feel the pos-sibility of crossing that pain to reach the other polarity, self-compassionate and accepting support.

To *Resignify* also means to recognize the resources you can depend on, to know what motivates and fortifies you and to stay in touch with that source. You identify more with what it brings you and with those priorities. Also, you can let go more easily of whatever drains your energy and diverts you from your purpose, including certain people in your life.

To *Resignify* means being in the present with the possibility of imagining a free future, regaining the sense of control over one's life and the answers you give to the unpredictable. Like the ideogram of the Chinese emperor, you manifest a coherence of feelings, thoughts and actions, all aligned with your sense of personal mission. There's no room for arrogance. There's only humility and surrendering to what is.

I'll add something more. It's like a muscle when you exercise. You can strengthen yourself in such a way that, even though you sometimes hit low or painful states, it's easier to look at situations differently and make adjustments organically. Depending on how you look, you can always find a bonus behind what hurts.

And do you know how you know you're doing well? Your body expresses it through relaxation, peace and a total sense of well-being.

Finally, to *Resignify* is to have more awareness and appreciation of your health. We take it for granted too often. Then it takes a powerful, painful event for us to begin to really value not only our health, but life itself. Even though it's imperfect, we can learn how to thank life. In fact, the reason you can feel that things aren't perfect is because you're alive. And if that's so, there are always possibilities.

CHAPTER 33

CONTEMPLATIVE TOOLS

"When we reach the edge of the door we can pass through or stay outside. If we do not enter, we will not return to that threshold, if we pass through, we will never lose our way. "
— J.L PADILLA

Over the past two decades, there's been a growing interest in the study and integration of contemplative practices as tools for health. They've even been formally adopted, enriching traditional medical and psychological practices. Since it's been shown that they affect happiness and well-being, the goal has been to apply these practices to enhance training in psychology and develop new therapeutic tools. This has also led to the development of new, more integrated and compassionate models of intervention.

Through mental training, combining contemplative practices and the latest advances in positive psychology, you can acquire the skills to fortify your psychological well-being. As with anything that's aimed at transformation and change, the keys to success are regular practice and dedication.

I want to share several practices with you that have been transcendent in my life. I don't consider myself an expert in either, but they're my inner reinforcements, my soul food. For years they've been daily companions. Having my space of stillness and silence, just breathing and focusing, is partly what allows me to go through the day being captivated and seduced by all the stimuli around me. Education is generally more focused on external knowledge, on the rational and the intellect. Thankfully, I had a lot of freedom at home and in my first school to develop other areas and begin my spiritual sowing. Even so, one of my biggest challenges has been to learn how to quiet myself in the midst of activity, external and internal noise and daily demands. Without a doubt, meditation has allowed me to participate in the world and live in it without feeling foreign or alien. It has allowed me to enjoy being earthy – a normal, ordinary person – while also having a sense of transcendence and my own inner space.

That intimate space belongs only to me and gives me an ongoing sense of orientation. Maintaining that center has allowed me to "have my feet on the ground and my head in the stars." This is a phrase I heard from a professor, Dr. Abate, at the beginning of my adult life. I believe he was actually quoting Theodore Roosevelt who said, "Keep your eyes on the stars and your feet on the ground." In any case, it describes what I want to express.

Like most people these days I have immediate access to the world. We're in the age of multitasking and instantaneous social networks, an era when no one even considers being disconnected. Presumably, just like you and many others, I perform numerous tasks and roles, sometimes with dizzying speed. I stretch time, hurrying from one activity to another, and always with more things to do. All of this is on top of my personality, with my tendency to always be doing something, plus having lots of interests and never wanting to miss anything important. I really don't know what I'd be like without the tools to center myself.

The moments when I'm sequestered in my own inner world are increasingly important and non-negotiable, even though I know I'm missing out on certain things. These moments have become a "prior commitment" that keep me from being always available to others. Still, it's curious to see that the time I've spent in that interior, separate space has actually brought me closer to many people and given me a deeper sense of my humanity. Taking more individual, quality time has allowed me to be more present the rest of the time. It's broadened my channel of compassion and sharing. And I'm still learning.

MEDITATION

I first encountered meditation in 1986. I began to practice and learn about it and I still consider myself a novice. Meditation is an art. It's a practice, discipline or technique for quieting the mind's dialogue through peace and inner stillness. It's for quieting the mind and transcending. As Shakti Gawain has said, meditation is a way to silence our "mental conversation" and connect with our deepest, wisest and most intuitive mind.[58]

Although many religions use meditation as a resource, in my opinion it's not a religious practice, nor does it belong to any one doctrine. Of course, it's an ancient practice central to the spiritual development of many monks and gurus and there's always been empirical discussion about the benefits of this practice. But more recently, thanks to neuroscientists, psychoneuroimmunologists and other researchers, there's been a special interest in the therapeutic application of meditation and in verifying its effects.

There are many methods of meditation, almost all of which speak of concentration and universal consciousness. The concentration brings attention to a positive image, our breath, or the repetition of a *mantra* (a repetitive sound), so our thoughts calm without resistance. It's not about wanting to push thoughts away, because the more you try to do that, the more they come. It's about not resisting and simply observing them, letting them come and go and gradually changing your attention to your purpose.

Meditation is very effective for self-observation, since it gives us a perspective disassociated from everyday reality while simultaneously helping us reach a higher consciousness.

In 2011, the Association for Psychological Sciences published the results of a study conducted by the University of Massachusetts in conjunction with the Bender Institute of Neuroimaging in Germany. This study concluded that meditating daily for 30 minutes over eight weeks generates favorable changes in areas of the brain associated with learning, attention, emotional management, empathy, stress and memory. There was also an improvement of intellectual performance and executive function and an increase in the grey matter in the brain.[59]

In 1991, a professor of Neurobiology at the University of California named Jack Feldman discovered the pre-Bötzinger complex, an area of the brainstem that contains neurons that are rhythmically activated with each breath.[60] It's a kind of respiratory pacemaker – though quite different from a cardiac pacemaker – and it's capable of a wide variety of different rhythms, such as when we yawn or during sleep. Mark Krasnow, a professor of biochemistry and co-author of a further Stanford University study relates that "this is not a region that simply provides air to the lungs, but these breaths are also associated with social and emotional cues." [61] Every time we inhale or exhale these neurons are activated and perform like a respiratory pacemaker. Stanford researchers also found that during meditation this region is considerably activated. So meditation not only helps us develop greater control over our breathing, it also helps stimulate a physical and emotional sense of well-being.

The heathy role played by the practice of meditation has been amply demonstrated through many studies and in many research papers. The practice has been surprisingly effective in strengthening the immune system and reducing the "inflammatory cascade." It can also have a favorable effect on obesity, cancer, cardiac disease and depression, as well as other diseases. So it's an excellent complement for physical, mental or emotional health situations and these studies have helped more people approach it with greater confidence.

Some other benefits of meditation that have been demonstrated include development of self-observation, development of intuition, greater trust in inner wisdom and the sense of spiritual being.

An excellent step, in my view, is the introduction of meditation as an addition to physical or psychological treatments in medical and healing centers. In some places this practice is now recommended for people with depression, anxiety and fibromyalgia, as well as for cancer patients both during and after chemotherapy. Everyone can meditate, even children.

Meditation invites you to meet your most intimate, serene and unknown side. Regardless of what technique you choose, it's a way of focusing and inducing yourself to investigate your inner nature, to reconnect with the best of you and with the art of living well in a fresh way. To quote the popular writer, Alan Cohen, "If you want to find God, hang out in the space between your thoughts."

Here, in list form, are some of the benefits:

• Strengthens the immune system
• Increases available energy levels
• Lowers blood pressure
• Reduces pain from tension: headaches, joint or muscle pain, ulcers

- Improves insomnia
- Decreases blood lactate levels, reducing anxiety attacks
- Increases the production of serotonin which, in turn, improves one's mood
- Relaxes the mind and decreases negative thoughts
- Improves and increases focus and mental clarity
- Helps emotional stability
- Stimulates creativity, intuition, self-observation and alertness

Meditate regularly to get your benefits and make it part of your daily routine. Reading about its benefits won't help you, but practice will. Try it!

MINDFULNESS

Mindfulness has its origins in meditation and, similarly, one of its main objectives is to connect us with the present. It's a term that's become fashionable and seems valuable as a way to adapt a meditative practice to the modern era. Mindfulness has also been enriched by new contributions from research and experimentation. So it's both a simple practice and a renewed one.

The term *mindfuless* was coined by Dr. Kabat-Zinn, a physician, molecular biologist and researcher at the Massachusetts Medical Institute. His research and development has focused on health and clinical applications of mindfulness training for chronic pain and stress-related problems or disorders. This includes studying the effects on the brain of a technique called MBSR (mindfulness-based stress reduction). MBSR measures how the brain and the immune system process emotions, particularly under stress.[62]

Kabat-Zinn has taught mindfulness to groups from a wide variety of professions. "Mindfulness," he writes, "is "deliberately paying attention to the present moment, with acceptance"[63] It is seemingly quite simple but requires serious practice to keep our attention focused on everything we feel or that happens to us. Yet the goal is simply observation, without judgment, reasoning, calculation or speculation. It's about living in the present, open and receptive. Mindfulness invites you to become aware of how you relate to experience in the present moment. It's being here and now, paying attention and nothing more. And when you get distracted, you come back again to the present and try to remain as attentive as you can. No matter what you're doing, you can connect like this in an instant. You stop, you feel and you focus. Your full attention has only to do with what's happening in the present, which allows you to live each moment more fully. It's also a key tool for listening to the body. It leads you to explore the mind-body connection, as well as the role of thoughts, emotions, reactions and behavior patterns.

To be clear, the purpose of the practice of mindfulness isn't to go anywhere or feel anything special or retreat to a mountaintop or reach a sublime state. Kabat-Zinn, whose career has been dedicated to the development and expansion of this practice, describes it as the simple yet complex process of "expressly observing body and mind, allowing our experiences to unfold moment to moment and accepting them as they are." [64]

In this way, an ongoing disciplined practice gradually trains the mind toward calm concentration and attention. It cultivates an ability to realize what's happening as it happens. This helps to refine our inner observer and, in the exact moment of an experience, to realize more. This gives us the opportunity to change our relationship to our experiences.

Both meditation and mindfulness, allow us to transcend the limitation of the finite mind to access another space, another universe. At the same time, they invite us to be in the here and now, discovering the magic of the present moment.

CREATIVE VISUALIZATION

I love and enjoy this excellent tool. I used to teach it as a part of my stress management workshops and programs. Over time it became a resource I use indirectly to facilitate other techniques. In 2003, after years of teaching these workshops and, to enhance my work as a facilitator, I decided to create and record several visualizations. I have them available in audios to help introduce people to this technique (though as of now they're only in Spanish). I also periodically listen to visualizations. Sometimes when I'm very tired and my mind is scattered I use them to help me re-center.

The mind works with images. Visualization is nothing more than the use of that ability we all possess to create a clear mental image of something, as if it were happening. We can use it consciously to create in a mental way whatever we wish to achieve, as if we've already achieved it.

By understanding some basic concepts about the functioning of the brain and our inner capabilities, you can use visualizations to record images in your mind that reflect what you want to attract. In the same way, creating such images can help you achieve physical and psychological benefits, such as a lessening of negative thoughts, nervousness, anxiety and fears and improving various diseases. You can bring to your body the serenity and mental tranquility you achieve with the practice of visualization.

Visualization is a very old practice, and actually, it's something we do naturally and spontaneously. The mind usually works by creating images and these constitute much of the content of our thinking. In visualization, the image is simply created intentionally, at a time of our choosing. And we can choose pleasant, positive images that provoke the psychophysical effects we desire. We can provoke emotions and sensations as if they were real. This makes visualization an effective anti-stress technique.

According to Dr. Karl Pribram, director of the neuropsychology department at Stanford University and a world-renowned authority on the functions of the brain, the power of our thoughts, ideas and words is largely due to the fact that they're translated into images before the brain can interpret them.[65] Images then, have great influence over our emotions, our actions and our organism.

The brain can also draw mental images, regardless of whether they make sense or not. The formulation of images depends on three conditions: your personal capacity to generate them, your own experience and your persistence.

The capacity for creating mental images and sensations is not the same in all people. As with any skill, there are those who exercise it more easily. But everyone can practice visualization. If you bring to mind places or moments you've experienced before, you can draw on your imagination or your experience. You can also create whatever scenarios you like, through creativity and fantasy. When you visualize something with the greatest possible level of detail, sensations are generated as if the scene were actually happening. For example: a moment of tranquility and peace by the sea, imagining the colors, the sun, the noise of the waves, the sensation of the sand under the feet or the smell of salt.

RELAXATION PRACTICES AND CHILDREN

In 2011, I published my first book, *Los Colores del Amor (The Colors of Love)*, and it's a work dedicated to children. It's actually an instruction manual for parents, guardians, teachers, therapists or adults who are responsible for children, and it's about the process of guided relaxation and visualization. The book is accompanied by an audio CD with three guided relaxations, designed for children to periodically listen to, after an initial hearing with an adult. One of my big dreams is that the relaxation and visualization practices for children that I share in this book are officially introduced in schools as part of education. I believe that if these practices were introduced to children throughout the world, it could help lay the foundations for a planetary change.

My goal in writing *Los Colores del Amor* was to find an effective and simple way to introduce children to visualization and to give them a resource that supports them in managing the challenges they face. The book also seeks to help them optimize their cognitive, intellectual, creative and bodily potential, to positively affect their general health, school performance and behavior.

Of course, if the parents don't get involved and consider it important, the book is not likely to really succeed.

As a way of continuing to support children, I also designed a simple program I called Aliento Kids. This is a workshop where we teach relaxation techniques, guided visualization, mindfulness, concentration techniques, brain gymnastics and conscious breathing exercises. The workshop has succeeded thanks to two psychologists, Jacqueline Bobea and Rosa Milagros Rojas, who've enriched it with their own experiences and who work lovingly, directly with the children.

In 2014, I created another more involved and elaborate program named after the book and called Taller Creativo Los Colores del Amor. This workshop offers children a comprehensive and creative program in which different techniques of relaxation, breathing, brain gymnastics and concentration are taught consciously and dynamically through plastic arts, theater, dance and play therapy. The curriculum is based on principles of mindfulness, systemic pedagogy and creative pedagogy. Like Aliento Kids, this program is periodically offered at Lunavital.

With the support of our Luna Life Foundation, we're now in the process of introducing these tools to children who have cancer through a project we call Libélula (Dragonfly). The hope is that changes in emotional well-being for these small patients will be translated into changes in their body biochemistry that favor the immune system, bringing better therapeutic results and overall health.

ACTIONS FOR A R.E.A.L. LIFE

MINDFULNESS:

Wherever you are, at any time of the day, just stop and focus on your breathing. With open eyes, inhale through your nose and exhale through your mouth. Breathe deeply, engaging your abdomen. Focus on the sound and rhythm of breathing. Be prepared for your thoughts to drift. Don't fight it and don't blame or judge. Just bring your attention back to your breath each time you realize you're distracted. This basic meditation technique helps restore your mind and brings clarity and peace.

Take a moment to focus only on your heart. Feel how the muscle expands as you inhale and contracts as you exhale. You're breathing with your heart. Continue for a bit. This simple exercise in full attention can help if you're distracted in any way. It helps you return to you.

VISUALIZATION:

Go to a quiet place. Relax and breathe deeply. Soft music and/or an aroma might help.
Now visualize a clear, detailed image of a calm, beautiful natural place. It could be someplace you've actually been or just an ideal place you imagine. Notice the colors and textures. Add any elements you like: water, flowers, sand, trees, sky. Sit in a corner of that beautiful, peaceful environment. Remember to breathe evenly and keep your mind open. Don't judge whatever else might appear. Also notice what's happening in your body. Enjoy this for as long as you like or until it feels like enough. Say goodbye to this special place and slowly return to the present, becoming more aware of your body and where you are. Make gentle movements with your hands, feet and head and open your eyes.

CHAPTER 34

CHOOSE TO LIVE IN GRATITUDE

"Gratitude is the memory of the heart".

— LAO TSE

Gratitude is a healing force that helps us to focus on what we have, including however we're able to function in the present. It help us focus on our opportunities and achievements and can bring us closer to what we want. It's the inner force that connects us with our true nature and helps us to awaken a sense of personal fulfillment. When we bring gratitude to the body we connect to the present, the here and now, and the fullness of experience.

Some time ago, I set out to live in a grateful frame of mind. It's been a challenge because I sometimes separate myself from that purpose. But then I return to the center where I can find my own light and more and more I'm able stay in that special resonance. Personally, I feel it's like a state of complicity with life. I feel that being alive is a great privilege and that alone deserves my total gratitude. By focusing more on what I have, as opposed to what I lack, I've been able to better appreciate the details of everyday life and the abundance of small miracles. I lose myself less, find myself more and feel lucky for it. I give thanks for my health, for being able to contact the world through the senses. I can see, hear, feel, touch, talk, eat, laugh, love; I have so much, the list is endless. By living this way, I've noticed that my complaints have greatly diminished and my energy is stronger and more consistent.

I'm not saying that living in gratitude requires that everything be perfect or just how we think it should be. There are always easy moments when we spontaneously feel thankful because we're happy, because we get what we want. But as you well know, we also face challenges and unfortunate, complex times when things are not what we expected. Then it's more difficult to maintain a grateful attitude. Like you, I've been there many times. But in the midst of cancer, staying focused on gratitude for being alive and for all of my resources and opportunities was truly essential for keeping my energy high and overcoming the disease. Remaining thankful is what kept my immune system on my side.

Regardless of the circumstances, this state of gratitude is realized when we're tuned in and able to see the learning behind everything that happens to us, in hard times as well as easy ones. It comes when we can see in each of life's potholes a lesson to learn, when confronted with an illness we can learn to see a teacher. It comes when pain becomes a valuable element and our mistakes become experiences that help us to do better or at least different next time.

Gratitude definitely heals. Because by being thanking from the heart we modify our energy, we change our body's biochemical state and our defenses improve. The stress that damages the organs and systems is transformed into well-being.

We've discussed how the heart is not only a mere pump that receives and drives the blood but also has a built-in nervous system through which it communicates with the brain and the whole body. The heart can send powerful orders of

healing. It creates an electromagnetic field that sends signals to all the cells of our body and even further, around
our entire physical periphery. Tuning in with the heart
through a positive emotion like gratitude – with its heartbeat, energy and intelligence – changes the electromagnetic
field, generating a more harmonious state in which the
work of our biological systems is more synchronized.

Our first relationship model is established with our parents and all of our other relationships proceed from there.
That model creates what's been called our *inner image*,
which stays in the unconscious. Our tendency is to repro-
duce that inner image or unconscious vibration in the other
relationships we form throughout our lives. The same thing
happens with gratitude.

Living in a state of gratitude is also a process. It's
achieved when we practice and feed it. It's achieved when
we decide to see grace in all that happens to us, even if we
don't understand it in the moment.

To live in a state of grace is to live from a more spiritual
dimension, to experience life's processes from a more loving vibration. Everything that happens is embraced in our
heart and its warm joy. It is liberating and expansive. We
can turn difficult situations into allies, teachers and friends.
Be thankful then, for those moments that teach us through
each experience. Many times, in the face of failures and de-
feats, our accumulated learning can take the form of new
skills, a clearer vision, greater peace and more confidence.

When the heart is filled with gratitude we live life from
abundance. We meet situations with the certainty that we
have the resources to face what life brings us, even losses,
sorrows and pain. We attract abundance by wishing that
nothing be other than it is in that moment, by simply saying, "Yes, Thank you!"

Bringing this gratitude to the level of the body and
health is about directing our gaze toward the blessing of

being alive, whatever ailment or discomfort we may have. Even if some part of the body is sick or doesn't work well, we're still alive and we still have a chance to change. To live in gratitude is to live in celebration. Celebrate the miracle of life and live in communion with the Immeasurable Great Force that makes everything possible.

ACTIONS FOR A R.E.A.L. LIFE

Close your eyes and imagine yourself in front of your parents. See them as large and you're small. Be present and connect with your inner light. Now, simply say. "Thank you." Do this daily for 21 days. It's simple and powerful.

Breathe with your heart, as I've previously explained. Tune into the heart's gratitude and give thanks for the life that you've been given. Give thanks for all of your family, your relationships, community, work, opportunities for growth, for your food, for nature. For everything that occurs to you, say, "Thank you."

Give thanks to your body. Realize that despite whatever limits, pain, diseases, injuries or discomfort you may have, you're still alive. Thank your body for being there for you, for surviving ins spite of you ignoring it's needs or whatever mistreatment you've sometimes given it. Thank your organs, the healthy and the sick. Thank each of your cells, all your tissues and all that flows through your body. You're here! Give thanks when you rest, or when you bathe. Give thanks during a massage or any other treatment, or when you apply a cream or an oil. Keep giving thanks.

Give thanks for nature, a source of energy that feeds, renews and cleanses you. It provides the perfect habitat for your life. Give thanks for the sun, earth, sea, trees, rain . . . for all that surrounds and sustains you.

Make a jar of gratitude. Write down things you're thankful for on little pieces of paper and put them in a jar. You can do this for a particular time or situation or start in on the first day of a new year and add a new note each day. At the year's end empty the jar and read 365 reasons for being thankful. It's powerful. Be creative and look for other ways to be attuned to gratitude.

The miracle
occurs in the
heart
when we
surrender
to the
mystery

RAQUELLINA LUNA

EPILOGUE

While working on this book, I rediscovered a story I wrote some years ago. It was a nice surprise because I didn't remember I had it. It's a tale of a caterpillar who becomes a butterfly, a metaphor that's been widely used. But for me it still beautifully represents a human being's process of transformation. It never loses its resonance and always leaves a good feeling. I had just rediscovered the story when I was diagnosed with thyroid cancer.

You may or may not know this, but the thyroid has two lobes and is shaped like a butterfly. It's in the neck, the bridge between the head and the rest of the body, which represents the bridge between the brain and heart. It's in the throat, from whence we express our thoughts and feelings through words.

This connection between my butterfly story and my cancer came to me three days after my diagnosis as I was sitting in meditation. It framed many things for me and moved me in a powerful way. After the feelings had settled into place, I felt like I could access a new level of personal work. I felt invited to silence, to return to the caterpillar experience inside the dark and lonely cocoon, to travel a silk road to another state of consciousness.

I hope that you discover your own path on the butterfly route: your R.E.A.L. path. Live every part of the process, every step. Your story is your wealth. Your experiences are your legacy. When you're a worm, crawl and let yourself be surrounded by darkness. Surrender. Feel in your own intimacy the transformation toward that intermediate state, the time of the chrysalis. Then let the next movement emerge and surrender to it patiently. Everything you need is inside. The love of Providence sustains you. Trust and follow, because the moment always comes for your most sublime expression, when you take flight!

Heal, recognizing and celebrating yourself. Celebrate your journey. Celebrate that every day you have something new to learn, that every second is an opportunity to choose, to get up, to continue. Thank and celebrate every moment you breathe. Celebrate having companions that inspire and enrich your journey. Recognize and celebrate your body, your health, your family, your clan. Celebrate your learning and curiosity, the privilege of being here, the divine in you. Dress up your festive heart and keep dancing at your own pace, at the same time pulsing with the heart of the universe and releasing yourself into God's embrace.

Embrace life, hug yourself. Love life and love yourself. Smile and live fully. Trust that everything that happens to you is part of the order of the universe. Every encounter is sacred, every moment is destined for your growth and is miraculous. May your light be present in everything you do and may all you do be at the service of something greater.

Bon voyage!

ACKNOWLEDGMENTS

To life, as it was given to me through the best, Marcelino and Raquel and, through them, to all who preceded them.

To my family, always present in everything I do, sometimes silently and always in close support.

To all my teachers, mentors, friends and supporters from whom I've received so much in this process of searching and meetings.

To the Lunavital team from its founding until today. Thank you for teaching me teamwork and for helping me realize one of my big dreams.

To all my patients. Thank you for trusting and for allowing me to do my part in the best way I could, and above all, for learning.

To Rosa Milagros who supported me by reading the first draft and making the first corrections. They were long hours of typing.

To Roxana, my first editor, proofreader, counselor. Thank you for going further, for allowing me to make beginners mistakes and continue with courage until the end. Your patience and rhythm taught me a lot.

Isaiah, thanks for your enthusiasm. Thank you for reviewing my writing and giving your wise recommendations, aligned with my purpose. You are always there.

Juan, thank you for believing in my work, making others believe in it and creating loving bridges of collaboration.

Julissa, thanks for our meetings full of sparkle, freshness

and youthful inspiration. Thank you for interpreting my R.E.A.L project with your art and bringing it to the book through your beautiful illustrations and the final design.

Edward, my traveling companion, support, advisor, critic and enthusiastic supporter all the way. Thank you for putting not only your love at my service for this project, but also your wisdom as a writer. Thank you for your criticism, for your suggestions. You leave me encouraged to continue learning.

To my lights and shadows, which have allowed me to find my R.E.A.L. path.

APPENDIX I

SPECIFIC REFERENCES FOR PARTS OF THE BODY
A physical symptom is an opportunity to make us aware that an area in our life needs attention. Here are some observations from a variety of sources that may shed light on the corporal topography of a condition:

The Head
The head symbolizes the principle of authority and order. It relates to the subtle, the abstract, the mind, the ideas, the ability to imagine and project. It symbolizes the masculine, the father and all the male ancestors.

The head is the center of communication and is linked to individuality. When there are difficulties or illnesses of the head, often there are conflicting thoughts or conflicts with authority, spiritual life or personal growth.

There are various causes of headaches. They can come from stress or the effort and tension to be "up to par" or to "get with it." As the head represents the self, headaches can also be linked to low self-esteem, as when a person is labelled as not being this or that or not smart enough. Likewise the cause can be too much pressure, as in the case of a perfectionist trying to will a thing to happen that's beyond their control. A headache could manifest expressions like "I just lost my head," "What a headache!" "I'm being hard-headed," "I'm up against a wall," "I'm between a rock and a hard place," "This isn't what I had in mind," "I lost my head," and "I feel like my head is going to explode!" This last expression is often from built-up emotions or fear of the judgment when one has to "be the head" or take on leadership or to be the person in charge. Issues with the head may also be the result of an over-effort to understand everything and a rush to answer all questions.

In Psychogeneology it's been observed that tumors in the head or the brain, often have to do with secrets hidden in the family tree.

The Face

Facial expressions are often the purest expressions of emotional states. The face is associated with identity, the image. The face also has a relationship with the capacity to be responsible in the face of things and to "face the music."

The Eyes

The eyes relate to our capacity to see, to look and to communicate. Through the gaze, we express emotions. "The eyes are the mirror of the soul" and can express love, anger, fear, pleasure, seduction, surprise, indifference, sadness, joy.

Together, the eyes are masculine in character. The right eye is the intellectual, the rational, and relates to the external self and how we think others see us. The left eye is that of the heart, the deep eye, that of receptivity. It relates to the inner Self and how we see ourselves.

Vision problems are linked to not wanting to look or to "turning a blind eye" to something. At the energy level, in TCM, the eyes correspond to the energy of wood and relate to the liver and gallbladder. In addition, they're emotionally linked to anger, irritation and rage.

The Ears

They are related to the maternal (receptive) lineage. Deafness can represent something we don't want to hear.

- **Left ear.** Relates to "inner listening," to the need to be in touch with our beliefs and feelings.
- **Right ear.** Relates to the outside, to hearing outer events and circumstances in relation to actions.

The Nose

The nose is associated with intuition. It's the part of the face most projected forward and it points to the outside world. Our sense of smell, like our hearing, still works during a coma, and smell is the first sense to detect danger. Nose problems which affect the sense of smell are related to something that "stinks," both literally and metaphorically. In the latter case, this can also be in response to a sense of danger, insecurity, anguish or restlessness, or just not wanting to "stick our noses in."

The Teeth

They're associated with aggressiveness, vitality and strength. Dental problems can be related to lack of expression or to repressed aggression. Sometimes they reflect a difficulty with biting into something, applying ourselves or achieving a goal. Dental problems might signify that a person doesn't feel they have the right to be aggressive, they don't allow themselves to be critical. The teeth are held by the jaw and so also relate to willpower and strength. They often represent the degree of rigidity in our perception.

Throat

The throat is the channel of expression and creativity. It has a triple function: breathing, speech and swallowing. Therefore, three different issues might be experienced:

- **Throat closed.** Feeling forced to do or say something and resisting it.
- **Difficulty swallowing.** A situation, person or food that's "tough to swallow."
- **Difficulty breathing.** A struggle to commit to life, to aspire, to live with gusto, to enjoy.

Fear, repressed emotions or stifled creativity can be hidden behind tonsillitis. It can also reflect anxiety or the sense of being mute. Many throat problems respond to an inability to assert ourselves and ask for what we need. They might also signify a regret that you said something you didn't mean.

In children, tonsillitis can be related to not being able to get affection from their parents and feeling powerless. Children might feel they have to earn the love of their parents by being good and doing exactly what their parents want, or getting good grades. They have to fight for love. In this way, they feel they can't just be themselves. They're the classic "perfect children."

The Heart

In TCM, the heart is the emperor, who channels all emotions. It represents love and the joy of living. The heart is a pump allowing joy to circulate with love throughout the body. When we deprive ourselves of love and happiness, the heart shrinks, it hardens and cools and as a result our circulation slows down. Chest pain or a heart attack can result.

A heart problem can relate to emotional problems from the past, prolonged lack of joy, tension and stress. It can signify repressed aggression through excessive self-control. Heart problems are also linked to conflicts of self-esteem because the person can't defend their territory, whether real or symbolic (the family, home, the couple, the children, work, money, etc.). Many people with heart disease didn't listen to their heart. They've shut their hearts or let them harden so they no longer open and simply break. Heart disease and associated problems can also relate to a lack of self-love.

Lung

The lungs open us to our environment through exchange and communication, the giving and receiving. The lung signifies freedom and also union with all life as it maintains its rhythm with nature, flowing permanently (in respiratory rhythm). In TCM, the lung relates to metal and emotions of sadness, nostalgia, melancholy, longing, depression and mourning.

The respiratory system is dominated by notions of space, freedom and security. When these needs are not met, respiratory symptoms can appear. Respiratory problems translate into conflicts between what's given and what's received or in feeling a lack of space: "I hardly have room to breathe!" Lung issues can relate to a lack of inspiration in life or feeling unworthy to live fully. Conversely, when something or someone suddenly moves me, it "takes my breath away."

The Hands

Our hands represent choice. The right hand symbolizes rational choice. The left is the intuitive. The fingernails are our symbolic defenses. The thumb relates to intellect and concern. The forefinger (which points) relates to self, fear, father and authority. The middle finger signifies anger and sexuality, the ring finger to unions, commitment, alliances and duels. The smallest finger signifies family and secrets.

The Joints

Joint problems may be linked to a lack of fluidity or flexibility, resistance to change, excess control and poor adaptability. Pain in the joints, muscles and bones relate to a devaluing, a loss of self-esteem at work or in the family. These connect to someone saying "I can't do it," "I can't get there," "I won't achieve that." Of course, every joint can be looked at individually.

The Back and Spine

These are the system of sustenance and support. Spine problems often show a lack of feeling supported. They can reflect fear and the attempt to cling to old ideas, a lack of faith in life, a lack of integrity or someone who doesn't have the courage to follow their own convictions.

The back also relates to issues of rectitude, feeling over-burdened and/or undervalued. The unresolved conflicts of our past are often stored in the back. Back pain – and usually all osteoarticular (bone and joint) ailments – can signify devaluing conflicts. People with back, joint and bone problems can tend to be people who blame themselves when faced with a conflict.

In the lower back or lumbar region of the spine (which in the family tree signifies the parents) is the connection with our sexuality and creativity. As a crucial part of the support system, it's connected to feeling the burden of having to support yourself. Pain in this region can manifest emotional or material insecurities such as the fear of going broke, losing one's job or of having no support. This can apply to those who tend to take too much on themselves, dispersing their energies or those who "carry other's burdens," trying to save them.

The thoracic or dorsal region of the spine is the connection to our emotional part (and to our grandparents in the family tree). Mid-back problems can reflect an individual stuck in a past that remains a burden. This relates to conflict with one's "territory," or to feeling separate from one's clan, such as the feeling, "I can only count on myself." This region is related to the emotions and emotional guilt.

In the neck or cervical region of the spine we connect with our intellect (and the great-grandparents in our family tree). Issues here can signify a lack of emotional support, a feeling of not being loved. Here we find issues of withholding love, inflexibility, rigidity, stubbornness, control and imbalances regarding communication. This can be a person who refuses to consider other points of view or doesn't want to look back. This can also reveal imbalances with communication and control issues.

Carrying too much reveals an eagerness to appear powerful and industrious in order to compensate for feelings of inferiority.

The Shoulders

They are joints and also a place where we bear things, so they're related to support, protection, valuation and recognition and they represent the ability to carry responsibilities or burdens. Shoulder pain often has to do with feeling compelled to bear a heavy burden, as in "I can't bear it anymore," or "There's no going back," (so I'm stuck with this burden). And sometimes a shoulder issue comes from a sense of obligation, of taking on the problems of others or doing too much for someone else. On the other hand, the shoulders, along with the arms, can simply relate to doing things, to working. They also symbolize our ability to embrace and be embraced, in reality or symbolically.

The Hips

The hip is the fundamental joint for standing and walking. Hip problems can reflect a fear of making important decisions or of moving forward or losing balance. They can also reflect the experience of an emotional conflict in which it's difficult to sustain one's position, especially symbolically. They can signify a feeling of not being obeyed or followed, of losing authority, of being ignored or of losing importance, or being unable to stand one's ground. In young people, hip issues can reflect the struggle for something that's desired but can't be achieved, or a feeling of being limited, or not having permission.

The Digestive system

Conflicts affecting the digestive system are generally related to being able to both meet your needs (survival) or to seize the moment with new opportunities. They relate to ingesting, assimilating, and eliminating. They involve the relationship with the mother and everything in life we have to "digest." Many imbalances and conflicts with food and the digestive system are registered in the relationship with the mother at birth and at the oral stage.

In situations where food is or has been scarce, food can represent affection, safety, reward and survival. Periods of lack or emotional hunger in life tend to be filled unconsciously with food, especially in situations of separation, death, loss or lack of money. Symbolically, food can also help ease tensions brought on by economic, material or financial hardships.

- **Esophagus.** Relates to conflict that such as one when being unjustly taxed. It also relates to a sense of having to swallow something one can't accept.
- **Stomach.** Relates to problems associated with fear, anguish and anxiety. It reflects the ability to digest new ideas or new situations. As stated above, the stomach represents how we digest, absorb and integrate events. Gastritis for example represents irritation and anger at something or someone we can't accept. The stomach is also linked to the feelings of being deceived or entangled in a situation where one doesn't want to be.
- **Small intestine.** In general, it represents the absorption not only of food but also of our thoughts, feelings and emotions. The small intestine is associated with too much analysis and fear of scarcity. It also relates to the anguish of not receiving enough, conflicts of scarcity or starvation.
- **Large intestine.** It indicates an exaggerated eagerness to cling to the material and the inability to yield. It symbolizes the unconscious. Constipation can mean we're afraid to expose the contents

of the unconscious. There may be a fear of loss. It symbolizes the attitude of letting things flow, of spontaneity and it also shows the conscious or unconscious desire to retain and to control.

The Kidneys
In TCM, the kidneys are said to regulate the element of water. They work on the balance of organic fluids, eliminating waste water through the bladder. They also harbor will and control fear. They control the reception of *qi*, in harmony with the lung. In *Illness as a Path*, Dahlke and Dethlefsen suggest that beyond external causes, kidney disorders indicate the need to release distress and fear. The kidneys represent coexistence and harmony. Kidney stones relate to the accumulation of issues the individual should have alleviated long ago, but their development has stagnated and become blocked.

The Knees
They relate to pride, submission, modesty and humility. They represent the ability to yield and release in relation to others. They also can indicate a proud and inflexible attitude that doesn't want to kneel to others. Falling on your knees is a call to humility, to abandon arrogance or pride in a given situation. Knees can also relate to decisions and forward movement in life.

The Legs
The legs connect with the ability to advance in life, with changes of direction, new experiences, and choosing to continue, to follow a path, to move forward. Problems in the legs can indicate a fear of moving forward or a refusal to continue in a certain direction. The hidden meaning has to do with having a fear of the future and thus not wanting to move.

The Feet
They symbolize the territory connected with brotherhood and bonding with the feminine. They represent the place where we stand and all the ways we allow ourselves to be nourished. Weak foot support (walking almost without making noise or on the toes) signifies a lack of rootedness, as if one doesn't fully commit to living. Walking with the toes pointed inward is often a sign of childish aggression. When the feet noticeably point outward, this can reflect the search for a place in the world. Foot problems in general merit a review of one's sense of safety, rooting, fears of the future and not moving forward in life, staying in the nest out of fear. Foot problems can signify moments of paralysis.

The Skin

The skin is the largest organ of the body and reveals a lot about us, especially our self-assessment with respect to the outside world. The skin represents the image that people have of themselves and their self-love. It's related to defenses, external contact, friction, relationships. Skin problems are linked to conflicts between our inner life and the world. They reveal stress, distress and a sense of feeling threatened. The skin can signify security and clan membership. It can show separation conflicts and conflicts with boundaries and borders. The skin helps us make contact with others, but it can also be a way to isolate oneself. The very appreciation of qualities, the ability to gratify ourselves and communicate emotions, is reflected in the translucency and brightness of the skin.

Uterus

The uterus is the seat of creativity and fertility. It's the first home for the future baby. So the uterus symbolizes home, a refuge and life.

From the viewpoint of psychogeneology, a woman's uterus stores the memory of the wombs of all the women in her tree. So for example a current problem with motherhood can have its root in a problem with the motherhood of her grandmother. Some uterine problems may be related to having had parents who wanted a male child instead of a female. They can also signify sexual abuse, or having the task of caring for the family of origin, especially siblings, or being raised with a compulsive neatness, or obsessive cleanliness and perfection. In general, a woman with problems in the uterus has difficulty germinating a new idea or project, she has trouble knowing the right time to act.

ACCIDENTS

Accidents are not coincidental. They translate unresolved problems and lessons that must be learned (often the hard way). They signify things that are forced and our resistance. Of course, one has to look at the type of accident. If it results from the inability to slow down or stop, it reads like a statement of stress. If it's the result of carelessness, it can show a lack of meaning. If it comes from inattention or "falling asleep at the wheel," it can indicate indolence and apathy.

APPENDIX II

99 NAMES FOR SUGAR

Here are some of the names the food industry uses to mask sugar. I encourage you to read and learn to interpret the nutrition labels on packaged foods. Remember, ingredients are listed in order of quantity; major ingredients are listed first. Each of these has the same basic nutritional value and health consequences of pure sugar. They're added to give food a more palatable flavor and/or a texture that also creates a pleasant experience, an experience you want to repeat. Sugar is addictive.

1. Agave juice
2. Agave nectar
3. Agave sap
4. Agave syrup
5. Beaver sugar
6. Beet sugar
7. Beetroot
8. Black molasses
9. Black sugar
10. Brown rice syrup
11. Brown sugar
12. Butter syrup
13. Cane honey
14. Cane juice
15. Cane juice crystals
16. Cane syrup
17. Caramel
18. Carob syrup
19. Ceratonia siliqua (or carob) syrup
20. Coconut sugar
21. Concentrated
22. Concentrated fruit juice
23. Corn glucose syrup
24. Corn honey
25. Corn syrup
26. Corn syrup solids
27. Crystalline fructose
28. Dark sugar
29. Date sugar
30. Demerara sugar
31. Dextran
32. Dextrin
33. Dextrose
34. Diastatic malta
35. Diatase
36. D-ribose
37. Ethyl maltol
38. Evaporated cane juice
39. Florida crystals
40. Fructose
41. Fructose sweetener

42. Fruit juice
43. Fruit juice concentrate
44. Galactose
45. Glazed glas sugar
46. Glucose
47. Glucose solids
48. Gold sugar
49. Golden syrup
50. Granulated sugar
51. Granulated sweetener
52. Grape sugar
53. High fructose corn syrup
54. Honey
55. Invert sugar
56. Isoglucose
57. Isomaltulose
58. Lactose
59. Malt barley
60. Malt syrup
61. Malta
62. Maltese sweetener
63. Maltodextrin
64. Maltose
65. Maple
66. Maple mixture
67. Maple sugar
68. Maple syrup
69. Milk sugar
70. Molasses
71. Panela
72. Panocha
73. Pastry sugar
74. Powdered sugar
75. Purging honey
76. Raisin sweetener
77. Raw sugar
78. Refined syrup
79. Rice molasses
80. Rice syrup
81. Rubber syrup
82. Saccharose

83. Sorbitol
84. Sorghum
85. Sorghum syrup
86. Starch sweetener
87. Sucanat
88. Sucrose
89. Sugar cane
90. Sweet corn
91. Syrup
92. Syrup syrup
93. Table sugar
94. Treacle
95. Trehalose
96. Turbinado sugar
97. Xilosa
98. Yellow sugar
99. Zilosa

Common products that often have lots of hidden sugar:

- Alcoholic beverages
- Bread (in molds or slices)
- Cereal (even "Fitness / Diet")
- Cocktails / Mixed drinks
- Commercial granola
- Cookies
- Energy bars
- Ketchup
- Low-fat products
- Milk
- Packaged juices
- Salad dressings
- Soda / Carbonated drinks
- Spicy sauces
- Yogurt

NOTES

EDITOR'S NOTE: Given that this book is primarily for the average reader, as opposed to academics or researchers, I've left Spanish references untranslated and simplified the online source references. (EM)

[1] Chopra, D., *La perfecta salud* (Santiago de Chile: Ediciones Javier Vergara, S.A, 1990).

[2] https://www.who.int/about/who-we-are/constitution

[3] Dahlke, R., Dethlefson. T., *La Enfermedad como camino* (Buenos Aires: Editorial Cúspide, 2004).

[4] Koval, P., *Medicina para el Ser singular con dolor persistente u otros problemas complejo* (Buenos Aires: Ediciones Incertidumbre, 2011).

[5] Castillo, C., *Ecos del pasado* (Caracas: Gráficas Lauki, 2005).

[6] Zammatteo, N., *El impacto de las emociones en el ADN* (Barcelona: Ediciones Obelisco, 2015).

[7] https://www.biologicalpsychiatryjournal.com/article/S0006-3223(15)00652-6/abstract

[8] Bombay, A., "The intergenerational effects of Indian Residential Schools: Implications for the concept of historical trauma", *Transcultural Psychiatry*, Vol. 51(3) (2014): (320–338).

[9] Hausner, S., *Aunque me cueste la Vida* (Buenos Aires: Editorial Alma Lepik, 2009).

[10] Hellinger, B., *El manantial no tiene que preguntar por el camino* (Buenos Aires: Editorial Alma Lepik, 2007).

[11] Hausner, *Aunque me cueste la Vida.*

[12] Champetier, B., *Constelar la enfermedad desde las comprensiones de Hellinger y Hamer* (Madrid: Ediciones Gaia, 2011).

[13] Engel, G., "The need for a new medical model: a challenge for biomedicine", *Science.* 196(3): (1977). pp129-136.

[14] Hamer, R. G., *Summary of the New Medicine.* Málaga: Amici di Dirk, 2000).

[15] Miller, A., *El cuerpo nunca miente* (Barcelona: Tusquets Editores, 2005).

[16] Pert, C., *Molecules of Emotion: The Science Behind Mind-Body Medicine* (New York: Simon & Schuster, 1999).

[17] http://www.emocionsalud.com/viacutedeos.html

[18] https://www.betipulnet.co.il/download/files/The%20Conscious%20Id. pdf

[19] Díaz, L., *La memoria de las células.* (Buenos Aires: Editorial Kier, S.A. 2007).

[20] Hamer, *Summary of the New Medicine.*

[21] Tolle, E., *El poder del ahora.* (Buenos Aires: Penguin Random House. Grupo Editorial Argentina, 2012).

[22] https://nanopdf.com/download/recopilacion-de-articulos-de-plano-creativo-psicogenealogia-centro-el-arte-de-sa_pdf

[23] Lowen, A., Lowen, L., *Ejercicios de Bioenergética.* (Málaga: Editorial Sirio, 2000).

[24] Schnake, A., *Diálogos del cuerpo* (Santiago de Chile: Editorial Cuatro Vientos, 2005).

[25] Ibid.

[26] Wattenberg, L., et al. "Effects of derivatives of kahweol and cafestol on the activity of glutathione S-transferase in mice", *Journal of Medicinal Chemistry*, 1987; 30(8):1 399-403.

[27] Dahlke, Dethlefson, *La Enfermedad como camino.*

[28] https://www.ncbi.nlm.nih.gov/pubmed/27810402

[29] https://www.researchgate.net/publication/309097336_Plant_Transgenerational_Epigenetics

[30] Ibid.

[31] Lipton, B., *La biología de las creencias* (Sevilla: Editorial Ariane, 2006).

[32] Zammatteo, *El impacto de las emociones en el ADN.*

[33] Blackburn, E., Epel, E., *La solución de los telómeros* (Barcelona: Aguilar, 2017).

[34] Ibid.

[35] https://www.ncbi.nlm.nih.gov/pmc/articles/PMC3635949/

[36] Blench, J., *El destino no está escrito en los genes* (Editorial Destino, Barcelona, 2012).

[37] Blackburn, Epel, *La solución de los telómeros.*

[38] https://www.ncbi.nlm.nih.gov/pubmed/15234599

[39] Blackburn, E., Epel, E., *La solución de los telómeros.*

[40] https://www.sciencedirect.com/science/article/pii/S1550413109003027

[41] https://www.jpeds.com/article/S0022-3476(17)30635-2/abstract

[42] https://www.researchgate.net/publication/322523841_The_fetal_programming_of_telomere_biology_hypothesis_An_update

[43] Rau, T., *The Swiss Secret to Optimal Health* (New York: The Berkley Publishing Group, 2007).

[44] https://www.ncbi.nlm.nih.gov/pmc/articles/PMC1931610/

[45] Hamer, *Summary of the New Medicine.*

[46] Shapiro, S., Carlson, L., *The art of science of Mindfulness* (Washington, D.C: American Psychological Association, 2009).

[47] https://pubmed.ncbi.nlm.nih.gov/26559246/#article-details

[48] http://eprints.hud.ac.uk/id/eprint/22884/

[49] Wynters, S. and Goldberg, B., *The Pure Cure: A Complete Guide to Freeing Your Life from Dangerous Toxins* (Berkeley, CA: Soft Skull Press Editorial, 2012).

[50] Reich, W., *Character Analysis.*(New York: Farrar, Strauss and Giroux, 1980 (3rd edition).

[51] López Rosetti, D., *Estrés, la epidemia del siglo XXI* (Barcelona: Grupo Editorial Lumen, 2013).

[52] Cannon, W., *The Wisdom of the Body* (New York: W. W. Norton & Company, 1963).

[53] Selye H., *The Stress of Life* (New York: McGraw-Hill, 1950).

[54] Ibid.

[55] https://www.ncbi.nlm.nih.gov/pmc/articles/PMC2742561/

[56] Selye, *The Stress of Life.*

[57] https://www.heartmath.org/

[58] Gawain, S., *Visualización creativa* (Málaga: Editorial Sirio, 2000).

[59] https://www.researchgate.net/journal/1745-6916_Perspectives_on_Psychological_Science

[60] https://www.ncbi.nlm.nih.gov/pmc/articles/PMC3209964/

[61] https://med.stanford.edu/news/all-news/2017/03/study-discovers-how-slow-breathing-induces-tranquility.html

[62] Kabat-Zinn, J., *Mindfulness en la vida cotidiana: como descubrir las claves de la atención plena* (Barcelona: Paidós Ibérica, 2009).

[63] Ibid.

[64] Ibid.

[65] Pribram, K., Ramírez, M., *Cerebro y consciencia* (Madrid: Ediciones Díaz de Santos, 1995).

[66] Dahlke, Dethlefson, *La Enfermedad como camino.*

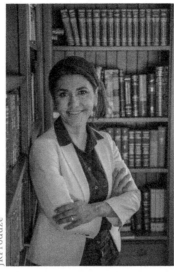

JRProduze

RAQUELINA LUNA is a doctor, psychotherapist, lecturer and author. Her practice is based in integrative medicine and complementary methods that support wellness, regenerative and preventative health. As a pioneer of integrative medicine in the Dominican Republic, in 1992 she founded the health clinic Lunavital in her home city of Santiago. She also recently opened an office in Brooklyn, NY.

Dr. Luna has presented courses, workshops and lectures for organizations and conferences throughout Latin America, as well in Europe and the USA. Beginning in 2010, she initiated *Bioencuentro,* a series of international health conferences, held in Santiago. Her work has been recognized with awards and accolades in the DR and internationally.

Dr. Luna founded Luna Life Foundation, which fosters community service programs in health and education in the DR and New York. In addition to *El camino de tu salud R.E.A.L.,* she's the author of *Los Colores del Amor,* a book for stress management in children.

WWW.RAQUELINALUNA.COM · WWW.LUNAVITAL.COM

EDWARD MORGAN (translator & editor) is a theatre director, playwright and educator. WWW.EDWARD-MORGAN.COM

Made in the USA
Middletown, DE
06 February 2021